From a wheelchair to walking, one person's Lyme story in Illinois.

Published by T.S. Banks

For

This book is dedicated to all the Lyme patients out there fighting for their lives and to the ones that did not survive. To my family that I love dearly that has seen me go through hell and back, and didn't give up on me, even when I wanted to give up on myself. You are my heart at soul. Also, for Jenny that tried to help so many others even though you were fighting such a hard battle yourself. We will meet again someday in Heaven. I promise you we will laugh and dance with all the other Lyme Warriors there.

Table of Contents

Chapter 1: Before the Illness

Chapter 2: Something is not right

Chapter 3:The bath, can I end it all?

Chapter 4: Lyme tests how many bands do you need to be positive

Chapter 5: Why must we continue to prove that we are sick

Chapter 6: Finding a good Lyme Literate Doctor

Chapter 7: The dark side of Lyme disease: Co-infections and Parasites

Chapter 8: Trying to help other's and explain this disease

Chapter 9: When you realize that you are not well enough to work

Chapter 10: Going Backwards

Chapter 11: Pain

Chapter 12: Not wanting to explain why you are not well

Chapter 13: New Doctor new hope

Chapter 14: Change is coming/Mercury removal

Chapter 15: Getting out of the wheelchair

Chapter 16: The Herxheimer reaction

Chapter 17: Cowden Protocol

Chapter 18: Things that I feel will help other summed up

Chapter 19: The Hospital and more understanding of Lyme in Illinois

About the Author

Suicide Hotline

Prologue

This book is written to tell my personal story of what I went through trying to fight for treatment from Chronic, or Late stage Lyme Disease in Illinois. Currently, I am not able to write my story alone, so my daughter is assisting me with it. The advice I give in these chapters are my own opinion. They should not be in any way taken for medical advice. I am not a medical professional or a professional writer. I am just a mom, a wife, and a sister that became sick and had to figure out how to get myself well. I wanted to share my story in the hopes that it may help someone else not have to go through six years of pain I had to endure. Thank you for taking the time to read my story.

Chapter 1: Before the Illness

I could work fifteen days straight, go to school at night, and still have dinner on the table for my family. I prided myself on being able to handle so much. I enjoy working, I loved school, but what meant the most to me was my family. I adored my kids, and there wasn't anything I wouldn't do for them. My husband helped with the housework, and even though life was crazy, it just worked for me.

At my job in accounting if there was an extra job to be done the boss knew he could count on me. I would even help other departments. I enjoyed working many hours, and I value myself as a good employee. Even though I worked quite a bit, when I was home I enjoyed spending time with my children. I would plan small things for us to do on the weekends, so we could spend quality time together. In those days it seemed I was always moving or going somewhere. It was impossible for me to know that soon my whole world would crash.

For me school was exciting, I was 36 years old, and I enjoyed learning. I loved the small classrooms at the community college, and when one class ended I was grateful to be able to enroll in another. I had met so many great people through school, that I knew when I graduated I will be sad. I came from a very poor family;

most women in my family grew up, got married, had kids, and that was their life. I felt school was a new adventure for me.

I had worked my way up from a warehouse job when my daughter was little. I found that I was good at collecting money for companies, and it was something I really enjoyed doing. I also found that at my age, the world had changed, and I needed a degree and experience if I wanted to continue to move up in my career. I had my daughter at the young age of 19. I married her father, and we also had a son in 2003. I was tough mom, but I loved my kids very much, and felt I was always very hands on mother. I would sit on the floor, and just loved playing with my children.

I found that I had to work very hard to move up in accounting without a degree. I had to work extra hours, take on more work, and prove myself constantly. I had grown up so poor that being able to make money and help my husband support our family gave me great pleasure. I loved to get up in the morning, most of the time I was the first one at work, because I enjoyed giving all I had to the company I worked for.

I had worked different jobs throughout my life, I started in a warehouse and one day they needed someone to file and answer phones. I had never done that type of work before, but I thought I would try it. I found that I had a good phone voice, and that I picked up things quickly. I went from a file clerk, to administrative assistant, to bookkeeper, then an accounts receivable clerk, with only a few computer classes. I wanted it all; the career, the family, the whole package. When my kids were little I felt bad for putting them in daycare, but I wanted to give them a better life then I had. I wanted them to not have to worry about things like food, and clothes for school. I grew up in a family of seven where money was very tight. We sometimes would go for days without eating much at all or living off things like a bag of chips and a 2 liter of coke. I made a promise to myself a long ago that if I was breathing I would do whatever it takes to make sure my kids had the best possible life I could give them. I never wanted them to endure what me and my four sisters did.

We were living in an apartment in Elmwood Park, and it was cramped, I decided I really wanted a house. My family had lost our mom in 2007, and I really felt a house would give our family a home we needed. I worked hard building up my credit, and I found an older fixer up house for us to move into. It needed so much work, but my husband and I worked hard and tried to make the house as livable as possible. I had brought the house from an older married couple, and the man was very sick. I was told he had MS, but at the time I didn't know too much about the disease to give it a second thought.

The house needed a ton of TLC, but I thought sweat equity, I was no stranger to hard work. We would do all the work ourselves: paint, put the new floors. I really didn't know anything about houses or fixing them up for that matter, but I figured we would learn as we went. My husband did have a background in construction, so I figured I would help him to the best of my ability and make this house a home.

Chapter 2: Something is not right

 I remember waking up about a year or two after buying the house and I was frozen. I could hear everything that was going on around me, but I couldn't move any part of my body. I laid in bed for at least 10 minutes before I could move at all. I thought that maybe it had something to do with an old back injury and decided to follow up with my primary doctor. At the time, the company I was working for was making lots of changes, and my doctor felt it had something to do with stress. She gave me some anxiety pills.

After the first incident, I began to experience odd things, like tingling in my face, hands, and feet. At first it was more of just an aggravation, and it wasn't very painful. The symptoms would come and go; I would get burning it my legs or my arms, my neck would hurt, different things that just did not add up. Around this time, I started having bad headaches, so bad that at times I had to stay in a room with no noise or light just, so I could rest. I went back to the doctor, had some more tests ran, and was told I had migraines.

My symptoms would go away, and new symptoms would appear. I started having stomach problems, I saw a different doctor, and I was told I had diverticulitis. It seemed like every few months I would get a different new symptom, and the doctor would tell me it was this or that. Then I started having lower abdominal pain, and I was diagnosed with PCOS, I had little cysts all over my ovaries. In 2012, my company that I had worked for almost 5 years was moving out of state, so I had to find a different job. I feel that that had put a ton of stress on me, and new symptoms started to appear.

I found that not only was my body burning or tingling, my hands were starting to go numb. I was having issues with my eyes blinking, or I was getting strange rashes. I had issues with my feet, they would burn, and my legs would get indents in them that I couldn't explain. I also found my mood was horrible; I would get bad mood swings. I had started a new job in April of 2012 and for the first few months everything seemed to be going okay. I was bit by a mosquito in July, and it was nothing out of the normal. I have had many bug bites over the years, as I loved to be outside, and sometimes the bug spray would not always work.

In August of 2012 I became very sick with what I thought was the flu. I went to the doctors again, I was told I had some type of flu, and just needed to rest. Around the third or fourth day of what I thought was the flu, when I stood up, I didn't have any strength in my legs, and I would fall right back down. My legs were very unstable, I had to hold on to the wall to walk, I felt so tired all the time, and every part of my body was hurting. I had horrible neck pain, and intense burning in my body.

I went back to the doctor; my family doctor was on leave, so I saw her partner. She checked me out and sent me over to see a neurologist. The neurologist ran an EEG of my legs, told me I had stress and sent me home. At this point I was having like an electrical shock in body. I would cry I was in such intense pain, and I couldn't find anything to soothe me. My family doctor finally was back at the office, and she ran some more tests on me. At first it was just a blood workup, checking for vitamins and such. She found out I had low vitamin d, and vitamin b. At this point my health had completely went downhill. I was having a hard time remembering things and at one point I couldn't spell my own name. Imagine being at work and not being able to remember why you called a customer, or who you were talking to.

At first it was the pain and throwing up that was causing me to miss work, then the seizures started. At this point I could no longer use my legs without the help of a cane. I would go through spurts where I would be okay one minute and fall down the next. I started having seizures at work, and it became pretty apparent that I was not getting better. The day I walked into my doctor's office on the cane, I think a light bulb went off in her head. She said I am going to test you for two things, because your symptoms are not normal. She ran a test for the West Niles virus, and Lyme disease. I had never heard of Lyme disease before and at this point I was desperate. On September 11th, 2012, I received the phone call that changed my life.

My primary doctor called me and told me I was positive for having Lyme disease. I didn't know anything about Lyme, and I thought finally I have some results. I started on three weeks of doxy, and boy was I in for it. I became so sick I couldn't walk at all and I was having a hard time just making it to the bathroom. When three weeks of doxy was up, I did not get any better, if anything I became worse. I called my primary doctor again, and I told her I was not getting better. It was then that I received the call from my doctor she had called me at home on her day off and informed me that she knows I have chronic Lyme. Also, that she could no longer treat me. She said that in Illinois the insurance companies would come in and close the offices down for treating Lyme patients longer then the three-week guidelines.

I was devastated, I was crying, and I didn't know what to do. She had given me a list of doctors in another state that she thought could help me. I spent the rest of the day calling doctors, most of the LLMD (Lyme Literate) doctors were so expensive, and I couldn't afford the first visit. At this time my sister had told me about her doctor that knew about Lyme disease, and my insurance would cover it. I went to see this new doctor with my test results in hand, explaining I had Lyme disease. At first, he said he could treat me, he knew about Lyme, and he could help me. He gave me some medicine for the seizures, and it only made them worse. When the medication didn't work he put me in the hospital for two days where they ran lots of test.

I had an EEG of my head done for the seizures, an Elisa test done, and many other tests. I saw many different doctors in the hospital those two days. I was first told my seizures were not real because they were not affecting my brain. Also, I was told my Elisa was negative so yes, I did have Lyme, but I cured myself. At the time I didn't know that Lyme hides in the tissue, and if you have had it a while, your body can stop making antibodies showing a negative test you still can have Lyme.

I was told I have Epstein Barr, and herpes 1 & 2. They brought in many different doctors and specialists. All the doctors seemed kind of aloof, like they didn't believe me, and that I was wasting their time. The worst doctor by far, was an infectious disease doctor. I was told he was a Lyme specialist. The doctor walked in my room, looked at me as I was shaking, and he said is this your seizures? I nodded yes, he said these are not seizures, you have muscle spasms. I explained to him about having the Lyme disease, and he said I have five minutes. When he left I was so upset, I just couldn't wait to leave the hospital. The next week, I went to get my results from the doctor, and I found out that this same doctor had written up a paper saying I needed mental help. His letter stated that I needed to be put into a mental institution, and that he did not believe outpatient therapy would help me. He never checked my legs or anything else. I used a cane, I could not walk, I would fall all the time, and he said I had mental problems. I remember feeling so upset and ready to give up.

When my sister's doctor couldn't help me, he sent me to a big hospital in downtown Chicago. I went to see two Infectious disease specialists that said I did not have Lyme anymore. After running more blood tests said I have inflammation in my body and sent me back to my primary doctor. At this point I had seen around 19 doctors; maybe more as I may have forgotten some along the way. It was horrible how I was treated when I told the doctors I had Lyme disease. I was told there wasn't Lyme in Illinois, and unless I traveled out of state I could not have it. I tried to explain to doctors that I used to live in West Virginia, but they didn't want to hear me. Around this time, I started doing my own research, I felt like I had to be my own doctor. I learned that most of my symptoms were related to the Lyme disease.

I felt desperate. I felt like the only doctor that believed me was my primary doctor, but she couldn't help me. I felt like I was failing my family, that I was failing my kids. I couldn't work, my last semester of school I was so sick I couldn't make it to class. I barely passed it was the worst feeling in the world. I still was driving a little at this point, just to the grocery store, and to the doctors. It came to the point where the seizures were so bad I couldn't drive anymore. One day, I was on my way to the store and everything started flashing, lights were everywhere. I couldn't see; all I saw was these big flashes of lights, somehow by the grace of God I managed to pull the car over. My husband had to come and drive me home. In January 2013, I lost my ability to drive. I felt like a complete failure. I had spent my whole life working for my house that I was losing, I was losing my job, my ability to drive, and at times I think I was losing my mind.

I was at the point where I wasn't working enough to pay my mortgage because I was too sick. Then we had found black mold in our home, and we couldn't afford to fix it. My primary doctor told me to just walk away from it. She said even if we spent thousands to fix it there was no guarantee that it would be livable. I started to get so sick at work; I worked for a company that manufactured metal racks that they painted on site, and I would throw up every day I was there. I spent more time in the bathroom than I did at my desk. The seizures I was having would make my whole-body shake, I couldn't control it, and afterwards I would have to use my cane because my legs wouldn't work. At first the seizures only happen at night, so I was still driving myself to work and school, but soon that would all change too.

I left work because I was having a seizure. My husband had to pick me up. I seized all the way home, my body just kept shaking and I was in a horrible amount of pain. I couldn't walk at all at this point; I had to use my cane. The day I left work I went right to see my primary doctor. I explained that I was getting worse, and she said that I could not return to work. That I needed to go on short term disability right away. So, when I went home I told my job I needed to apply for short term disability, and that day they sent me a letter stating I was terminated. I had never lost a job in my life. It was heartbreaking.

For the first time in my whole life, I didn't know what I was going to do. I was too sick to work. I was in pain all the time. I was having more complex seizures where I would fall on the floor. My whole body would freeze up, and I had to wait until my husband could get me up off the floor unless I could scoot myself to the couch or bed. I was desperate, I didn't know what to do, and I couldn't control my body. I felt like I was a prisoner in my own skin. It became to the point that I could barely cook a meal or put clothes on. I wore sweatpants all the time, or pajamas. I didn't have the strength to dress myself, or even brush my hair. I felt like I was losing my life.

Throughout this whole experience I saw so many doctors; over forty-five. I would beg them to help me. I would explain over and over I was in accounting, I was a student, and now I can't spell my own name. Some looked at me like I was just plain nuts, others said the same thing over and over; "We do not have Lyme Disease here.". A few just came right out one way or another and said I was crazy, mental illness, overworked, stressed or just overweight. It's so humiliating to go to the doctor with your loved one, that did not understand why you couldn't get off the couch, or out of bed, to have a doctor take them in another room and tell them your wife could stop this if she really wanted too. Yes, this happened to me.

I can tell you as a person, as a wife, as a mother, I felt defeated. I felt what is the point of going to another doctor, of trying to get help when they didn't believe me. At this point I sunk into a bad depression. I physically could not walk on my own, and I hated asking anyone for help. There were so many times I would have to crawl to the bathtub, or to the bathroom, stopping as I went because the pain was just too bad, and barely making it there to throw up from the pain itself. Other times I would just try to stand up and end up falling. I fell so many times I 've lost track. I told doctors this. One said well you have a gait disorder, another said possible ALS. I knew what that meant. I know what an ALS diagnosis would mean; it would mean that I was going to die. I would not or could not accept this. I needed my husband to believe me, I needed my family to believe me, I couldn't' do this on my own. It took some time, but they started to realize that I was telling the truth, and that everything that I was saying was true. My hand and legs would freeze up and start to curl, so my husband had to try and open my hands. He saw it happen, he knew there was no possible way I could do that to myself.

One of the worst experience I had I saw a supposed to be top neurologist in Elmhurst. I was really scared to walk in his office, I had so many bad experiences already, and I just didn't know what to expect. At this time, I was using my cane that my doctor prescribed me, it was one of those ones that you can fold up and put away. I had this one because some days I didn't need it as bad as others. Also, it had this thing on the bottom like an anti-fall device, it helped keep me standing. So, we walk in and he looks at my state medical insurance. I had lost my great insurance when I was terminated, and he said, "I am going to stop taking this insurance, they don't pay me.". Then he looks over at my cane and asks if we brought that at a discount store. I thought my husband was going to snap.

I should have stood up right there and walked out, but I was fighting for disability and I was told by the hospital that he was a good doctor. He looked over my file and said if people tell you nothing is wrong with you, then nothing is, it's all in your head. I took a deep breath and said I have a positive Lyme test. He said "Where is it? I don't have a copy of that". I knew full well he did, I has previously sent it to his office. He did some neurological tests that I failed and said that it's possible I had MS, or ALS. He did not believe I had Lyme. Yes, he was fired sometime after. I knew right then I was going to either must figure this out myself or I wasn't going to make it.

Chapter 3: The bath, can I end it all?

 I was fighting for my unemployment. Fighting the disability company that didn't want to pay me back what I put in. I felt like my life was pretty much over. I ran bath water I could barely make it to the bath, and I almost fell on the way. I remember thinking I had lots of bottles of pills; I could take one bottle, and just lay down in the bath and go to sleep. I sat in the bath, and I thought about it. I was so desperate. I had posted on the Lyme website before I took the bath how bad I was feeling. I was laying in the bath, and my phone went off, I had a new email. At my most desperate time, I received an email, and a wonderful lady from the Lyme website helped me so much; she told me I would get better, it would be a long road, but I would get better. That email saved my life that day. I had felt like I had failed my husband, I had failed my kids, and I had failed myself. For this Traveler, I will always be grateful.

I spent so much of my time researching on the internet. I met many great people that were in the same boat as I was. I looked for medical published articles and realized there were so many people around the world just like me. They had all lost mostly everything in their life; most of them even lost their partner. I was lucky my husband did not walk out on me. I mean I am sick daily, he must help me to the bathroom, there are times he can just hold me while I cry, while I shake. Also, my poor kids, they must pick me up off the floor, get my medication to help try to slow down the seizures. I have had people in my life give up on me, think I was crazy, but my husband researched and tried to learn how to help me. My kids never made me feel like I was crazy, even though they can't cure me, they tried to be understanding of what I was going through.

Since I was doing so much research I started looking at Lyme protocols. I could not get a doctor in Illinois to give me antibiotics any longer, so I had to find something that would help me. I found a protocol that seemed to be helping people, so I was trying it. It consisted of Cat's claw, Japanese knotweed, and a few other herbs. I researched daily, and I added to it as I went. Since I didn't want to take lots of pain medicine, I found that ginger was a natural pain reliever. I started boiling up ginger and drinking it each day. I also started taking detox baths that consisted of peroxide, and epsom salt. When a person has Lyme disease they need to detox the body because the die off the bacteria will leave so many toxins in our bodies, and we need to get rid them. On the new Lyme protocol, I started having a good day a week, it doesn't sound like much, but it was the only time I could get up out of bed, cook dinner, I could even dress up, and apply makeup. I had a little ray of hope.

Around this time, I started seeing another doctor. He was a different type of doctor; he was a natural path doctor. I still had insurance at this point, so I wanted to get as much use out of it that I could. This doctor was very smart and very overconfident, but he did not treat Lyme disease, he treated the whole body. He ran lots of blood tests on me and found out I had chemical poisoning; I was in worse shape than I thought. He said my body was in a chronic state, and I also was having problems with my glucose. I saw him for about a month. He did help me with eating better.

He had me stop eating gluten, and sugar. One day in his office he looked at my husband and said, "Your wife is going to lose weight, and leave you.". I looked at my husband; he looked like he was about to jump across the table and beat the crap out of this doctor. I knew at once, this was not going to work. He was not the doctor for me.

He wanted me to try this intense detox where I just drank a shake all day and was only allowed one vegetable. The worst part of the detox was that I had to come off my herbal meds for Lyme. I lasted three days, and my whole body had such a bad rash all over. I was a mess. The pain that set in would take my breath away. I thought for sure I would be in the emergency room again, it was that horrible. I called the doctor and explained I was too sick I needed to take my medication. He stated in the future I would need to do seven days of it off the medication. I knew then I had to find a proper LLMD, and a good one.

I had a few people ask me what Lyme is like; I want to explain what it's like for me. I had control of my life; I was outside all the time enjoying my life. I would laugh, and spend time with my friends, family, and the people I loved most. On days when the Lyme is at its worst I don't want to be around anyone. I feel like I am lost in my own body. When the Lyme makes me not be able to walk, I feel like I am in a tunnel, looking out at Life, but can't join in. I found that instead of having fun and being a happy person, I was upset all the time. I would cry at the drop of a hat. I felt insecure as a person, as a wife, and a mother. When I lost my ability to drive I felt like I lost part of myself, that Lyme took it all from me.

At times the Lyme gets in my mind; it makes me think things that are not true. It tells me I can't beat it, I should give up. It makes me paranoid and wants me to quit. I have been doing tons of research, and the people that don't die from the Lyme typically killed themselves. I was at that point a few months back, if it wasn't for an email, and the fact that I didn't want to hurt my family any more than I had already. I would of went through with it. At this point in my life, I started thinking about God, I was never a very religious person, but I felt there was someone here trying to help guide me. I started to pray at night, and in the day time, whenever I felt desperate I would ask God to guide me, to help me. I figured since there wasn't a cure, I simply asked him to make me strong enough to continue to fight.

The first year alone we spent at least seven thousand dollars trying to get me better. My husband did everything he could to try this or that, he started to research too. We ran out of money so many times, but I still tried to keep treating. I couldn't stop. I was afraid that if I stopped I would die. I saw what happened to my body when I wasn't killing off the Lyme. I became almost like a shell of a person. I was in there, but my body refused to work like my brain was turning to mush. I couldn't allow my body to get any worse, so whatever I had to do, I was willing to do.

I know firsthand how this disease can make a person feel like they are going crazy, heck sometimes I did go crazy. I have since made it my goal to help as many people as possible realize they are not alone. If we look at other people that have gone through Lyme treatment, some have had to be put into a mental institution because they really did lose touch with reality. This can happen and does happen quite a lot. I feel that this is because one the brain gets inflamed, and two, the brain is full of toxins. Our bodies are not able to fight off all the toxins, and it makes our whole demeanor change. I was constantly getting like what I can only describe as burning in my brain. I remember telling a neurologist this. She said that was impossible, brains do not feel pain. I am sorry. That can't be true. If you have Lyme, your brain feels pain.

I sometimes get these sharp, burning sensations as if someone is poking it with an icepick, and then it feels like water or some hot liquid is swishing around in my head. There are times when it gets so bad I will just cry and wrap my head in a heating pad. It took me a few years to realize that I had toxins in my brain, so I found a product by Sarah Jergians called antixiox 11 cns /pns. The herbs are made for the brain, and it helps detox. This product must be popular now because they sell it on amazon. In the past I had to special order it. Getting the toxins out of the body are extremely important if you're like me and your body can't detox on its own, you will need to find ways to help the process. It will literally help with some of the really bad symptoms.

Chapter 4: Lyme tests - How many bands do you need to be positive?

According to Dr. H all you need is one of these bands and you have Lyme.

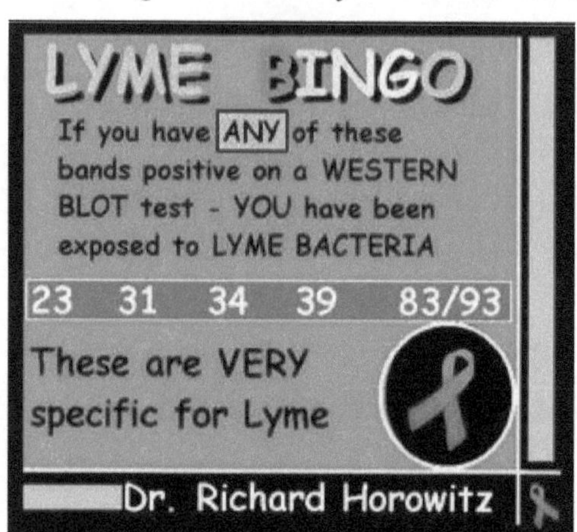

 The thing is I never had a bullseye rash when I was tested. I had one band come out positive, and that was band 23. I know people that have paid for five or six tests, have been sick for 15 years, and only after continuing to retake the test did it in fact come out positive by the CDC guidelines. Also, some of these tests are looking for antibodies, if we have had Lyme for a while our bodies may not be making them anymore. Another thing with these tests, the tests that are at the doctor's office only test for three strands of Lyme, the last time I checked there are over 100 different strands. Who is to say that the bug that bit you may not be from your region. It could have hopped off an airplane or off a suitcase from another country. There is really no way to tell. I also know people that have spent hundreds of thousands of dollars to get cured and have found there is no real cure. With the right medication and if caught early, you can have a normal life, but when the treatment is delayed our only hope it for the Lyme to go into remission. The truth is people are going to die, because the doctors are not trained to look for Lyme. Most of the tests are not accurate, and by the time it's found that we have Lyme it's too late for a quick fix. When taking the co-infection test I had five different co-infections. So, through this all I am not sure if it's the Lyme making me sick, the co-infections, or all the above. I started out with one band before I started treating; I have most of the bands now.

I was told I had many different things; from Lupus, to MS, to CFS, to Autoimmune disease. Through some of the research I have done, and talking to other people, I have found many people were not properly diagnosed, and had suffered for years. In my opinion if you are sick, and your doctor can't help you or does not take you seriously, it's time to find another doctor. It's almost like having an employee; if they are not doing their job, you need to replace them. Or if your car breaks down and your mechanic can't fix it, you find a different one. I have replaced my doctor over and over. I want a doctor that knows more about Lyme then I do. That is not going to charge me tons of money to tell me what I already know. I continued to look around, hoping to find a doctor that I felt could help me. We must be very careful mentioning the names of our Lyme doctors; even on the internet we don't use the doctor's' names. Too many of the LLMD have had their license taken away for treating us, especially in other states. We must protect them because they are the only doctors willing to help us in most cases.

If you are sick and have had test after test done, and the doctors can't find out what is wrong with you; do not give up. We must be our own support system or own advocate. The thing I had to learn through all of this is that I can't do everything. I had to learn to slow down, to enjoy the quietness, to listen to birds, and enjoy my kids. I had spent so many years running around I forgot to slow down and smell the roses so to speak. My life was rushing by, and I was just rushing with it. When I became sick, most days were spent lying in bed thinking. I had to reflect on everything I did in my life, some things I was not proud of, but I wasn't a bad person. I would ask God why he let this happen to me. Why am I to suffer, when so many other people deserved to be punished? I came to realize this disease is upon me to help me not hurt me. Yes, I must suffer, but maybe it's so I can reach out and help other people. Maybe I needed to slow down, because life is short, and I needed to learn to enjoy it.

Since the tests are not accurate, and many mainstream doctors do not treat Lyme disease, if you are sick you need to find a LLMD. In other words, Lyme literate doctor. A LLMD will most likely go off your symptoms instead of blood tests. In certain states this proves to be very difficult. I was told Illinois does not have Lyme. I'm sure lots of doctors tell their patients that depending on what state you are in. The thing is if a bird can carry a tick with Lyme disease, and a bird can fly, Lyme disease can be everywhere. I have talked to people from many different states and around the country and guess what they have Lyme disease. I do believe that it's not just the ticks carrying the disease. I believe mosquitos, and even fleas can carry the disease. Also, because bugs can carry Lyme, it can also carry other tick-borne diseases. I found that Lyme disease is the great imitator, and since most doctors are not trained to look for it, it goes undiagnosed. This disease is one of the fastest growing epidemics in the country, and around the world.

It gets to the point where you are so sick, so desperate, you will do almost anything to get well. I have found that people will play on this and try to take advantage of the situation. I have been emailed, stating they there is this or that cure, if I just buy this product. If there was a cure we would all be well, there isn't, this is a fraud. If you have Lyme disease you have already probably spent every penny you had, you may be facing homelessness, and there isn't anything you wouldn't do to get well. I know I have been there, I have tried crazy things that did not get me well. So, save your money, and do your own research.

Chapter 5: Why must we have to continue to try to prove that we are sick?

It's bad enough that we must continue to prove to our doctors that we are sick, and not faking it. Why do we have to prove to our family and friends as well? Not only was I told I needed mental help by one of my doctors, I was told this by others as well. I spent a lot of time thinking about this, and I can tell you I did not react very well to being told this. I feel like I am spending every day of every minute trying to have a normal life. I miss things that normal people without Lyme disease take for granted. I miss taking a walk or driving a car. I miss be able to think clearly, to not have to write everything down, and keep losing the notebooks. I miss not having to worry about if I have enough energy to go to the grocery store, or if I am going to have a seizure in the store and have everyone look at me. My words get mixed up, and sometimes just a comment from a cashier will get me so confused I fumble for words and feel stupid.

When I was driving I had to find a focus point to remember where I had parked my car. I had to make a list, so I knew what I was in the store for. I would get confused easy and find myself just standing in an isle not sure what I was trying to buy. I would get home and forget half of what I was buying, or I would buy too much of one thing, then remembering I had put it in the cart already. At one point I was washing my hands over and over, around the third time; my husband had to tell me I had just washed my hands. There are days when the whole day I do not make any sense, this worried me a lot. I couldn't hold a simple conversation. I know it upset my husband to see what I was becoming. I used to be this strong, successful woman, and now I was afraid to make a simple decision.

 I had people think I was making it up, I mean I looked fine, how can I be sick? I had a doctor tell me, I was not sick enough to have Lyme disease but too sick to have MS. Now how is that possible? I am to the point where I don't trust some doctors; I think a lot of them just try to push medication on us to get us out of their offices. If we had cancer, they would treat us, but since we have Lyme it must be in our heads. I don't understand why we are treated this way. A doctor's job is to help the people that are sick. I feel even if we had a mental issue, we would be treated better, then if we have Lyme disease. The doctors kept pushing me around and around, like I was piece of trash, not someone to take seriously, like I was stupid or crazy. I would tell them, I had a successful career, I was an honor roll student in all my classes, and I can't remember how to spell my name at times. How can nothing be wrong with me? How can it all be in my head?

I used to have a lot of friends. I was a very social person. Once I became sick some of the people that I considered my friend, started to avoid me. Maybe they felt my situation was too much for them or maybe they thought I was nuts too. I am not sure, but having people in your life, and then one day poof they are just gone without an explanation is devastating, especially as sick as I was. I had two people that I was close to just stop talking to me. I even asked if it was something I did, but I never received a reply. It hurt me bad at first because my circle was so small as it was, I couldn't get outside much. I had two people that I really cared about turn their back on me. It made me realize that I can't count on others to help me.

It's not like I had ever asked these two people for much, maybe some emotional support, but that what I thought friends were. I mean I am the type of person that if I find out you're in the hospital or having some surgery, I would cook dinner and bring it over to your house, so I knew you could rest and your family would have a good meal. My husband always said my heart is too big, and maybe that is true, but I would never do to other people what they have done to me. I would never stop talking to them because they became sick. I would try and be the best friend I could even if I didn't understand what was going on with them.

People reach out to me all the time online, and they tell me how their families, partners, even brothers and sisters just completely stopped communication with them because they have Lyme. Look, I know dealing with someone that is sick is not easy, I know it can't be easy to watch someone you love to go through something like Lyme. We need to remember as hard that it is for us to watch it, it's even harder for the person going through it. If you do some research you will find out so many people with Lyme show signs of mental illness like anxiety, depression, even hallucinations. I am going to be completely honest here; I have, and had, all these things. My anxiety was so bad I couldn't leave my house, if the doorbell rang I would go into a panic. When the Lyme hits my brain, I would get and still do get paranoid. Every single sound or light hurts my head. I get where sometimes I have random outbursts. I either get angry or emotional.

This is not our fault, but I had to learn how to handle it better. When I feel like I am about to explode I hide in my room or try to until it passes. Sometimes a herx can cause this, sometimes bartonella, a co-infection from the Lyme, and other times it's the Lyme itself. They call it Lyme rage, and if you're killing Lyme you're going to experience it at some point or another. People don't really understand it, and honestly, I don't understand it that much myself, but I can't control it. So, I needed to learn to try and control how I react to it. When I get like this I listen to music or watch a funny movie. I will tell you Netflix has been my best friend for years. When you're stuck in bed you must keep your mind busy. I was a huge reader. It was at this point where I couldn't read anymore, everything was going so blurry, so I started watching Netflix shows. I am a huge fan of comedies and romances. When you are sick and in pain if you can just get your mind off it for a few minutes or a few hours, it sure does help.

When you're stuck in bed, looking at the same walls day in and day out, it gives you so much time to think. I would stare out the window, I realized the seasons were changing, and I was no longer a part of it. It went from summer to fall, to winter, and I rarely ever made it down the stairs or outside anymore. I have a few people that I had worked in the past still be part of my life, but not like it was before I became sick. My friends became mostly only the people I met online, and most of them were sick just like me. We would kind of help each other get through the days and nights. Sometimes we would share information other times we would just share jokes or movies that we thought were good. Around this time, I found the Chicago Facebook site for Lyme. At first there were only a few people in this group, I looked at the group now and its thousands of people. Some people are in the same boat as I am. So many families have sick children, and do not know what to do to get them help.

I remember sitting in bed thinking that one day when I get better, I am going to do everything I can to make sure others do not go through this. No other children should watch their mother suffer day in and day out. No husband shouldn't have to walk away from their wife because she can't seem to feed herself, and her food is falling all over the floor. No one should go through 20 plus seizures a day only to be told that they could stop them if they really wanted to. I mean I begged doctors to help me, I lost weight, I did everything they told me to do, and guess what I couldn't stop the seizures, and neither could they. So, I started a Facebook page, Lyme in Illinois where is our cure, and I have been running that page for a few years now. People can reach out to me on there if they need help or just need someone to talk to. I have talked people out of giving up when the Lyme gets too bad. I understand it. I live through it.

Chapter 6: Finding a good Lyme Literate Doctor

We are now into April 2013, and there are changes taking place in the Lyme world. The state of Virginia has been under a 'Lyme war' so to speak. There are whole families being infected with Lyme disease. The people of the state are standing up, and senators are getting involved, a bill was passed about the testing for Lyme patients not being accurate. This is big news for all of us with Lyme. Thanks to a great lady that I have met through an online social website, a big protest in taking place in May for all of us with Lyme. There are many states involved and countries around the world. Maybe we are just all tired of being sick, and being ignored, maybe it's time that the insurance companies and doctors help us. We are not going to go away; we are all going to stand up for each other united, because of this horrible disease.

 I had spoken to a new female NP a few times on the phone, but just didn't have the money for the first visit. One of my sisters had brought a book for me about ways to help treat Lyme disease. This book changed my life; it talked about how oxygen would help put Lyme into remission, and how people are using rife machines. I spoke to her again, and she informed me that she had an ondamed machine and used oxygen for her patients. I was nervous about seeing another doctor, and her not believing I was sick. I didn't want to be let down again. My husband said if she doesn't help us we will keep looking until we find someone that will. At this point we were barely making it; my husband started working extra hours because the treatment for Lyme is very expensive.

We walked into her office, and it was not what I expected. She works out of her home, and the house just had a warm feel that I had never experienced in an office before. I explained to her what was wrong, and for once she did not make me feel like I was crazy. She is not one of those doctors that talks and talks, she listened to what I had to say. I felt comfortable with her. The first visit was three hundred dollars, because she uses two machines. She uses a Zyto machine to scan your body, and an ondamed machine to start to fix what is wrong. I admit I was skeptical at first. I did not tell her about some of my blood work because I wanted to know if these machines were real or if we were going to be taken for another ride again.

The machine started to pick up things that were wrong with me, things I didn't tell her about. It picked up things I knew I had like Epstein Barr, and herpes 1 & 2. It also picked up things I did not know I had like Rift valley fever (mosquito virus). I think the most amazing thing was when she asked me what was wrong with my back. I said nothing is wrong, I had forgot that years ago I slipped a disk in my back, the machine told her which disk was messed up it even showed on the report. My husband and I were both amazed. We started treatment that day. I started oxygen, and she used the ondamed machine to slowly start to help my body. She zeroed in on things like my immune system, my stress level, and finally viruses. She never makes me feel like I am crazy or not sick, she tells us of how some of her patients were getting so much better, and that gives us hope.

It was the first time in my life the doctor did not try to take me off my Lyme medication. She asked what I was on and added a few things to it. After the first visit, I made it five days without a seizure. Before I went to see her, I was having up to eight seizures a day. It was so bad I thought this is how my life is going to be until the Lyme takes my life.

I feel like I should explain what a Lyme seizure feels like to me. I usually get burning pain in my legs, this tells the seizure is coming. I try to lie down as soon as this happens, because if I don't I will fall. I feel burning all over, mostly in my left leg, and then it radiates all over my body. My head starts to feel like there is liquid in it swishing around. My arms and legs have what I called a tick, rapid movement all over at one time. I can't control it; I start to feel like bugs are crawling on my face, and I hear weird sounds in my ears. The light gets to be too much for me, as so does any sound. I shake all over, and my muscles feel like they are being zapped with electricity. The only thing my husband can do it rub my leg or my arm, then my whole body freezes up. I can't talk. My vision is very blurry. I see in double, and sometimes triple vision. This can last anywhere from five minutes to hours at a time. When the seizures are over, I am exhausted.

 So, when this doctor asked me what I wanted to work on first, I said the seizures. I need help with the seizures, and the pain. I had so much inflammation in my body my body would turn red. I have tried everything I could think of to take the pain away; the only thing that has really helped me is heat. There are times I take up to five baths a day. I would just sit in the bath, and cry, and beg God to help me. On the outside I looked just like everyone else, but on the inside, I was a Lyme infested mess.

After a few weeks of treatment, I am starting to see improvement. I can walk outside to the corner to walk my dogs, this would have been impossible a few months back. I can stand to cook dinner, and not fall. I still must rest quite a bit because I tire so easy, but I feel that I am starting to get my own self back. I am always doing research, seeing what is working for people and what is not. I started adding to my protocol; like oil of oregano, detox tea, and teasel root. I am seeing good results by trying different things, mixing it up so to speak. I figure since the Lyme is so smart, I must keep going after it from all different directions.

I can't find words to explain how it felt the first time I could play a ball game with my son. For the last year there were times I had to scoot to the bathroom, and I found my legs were working again. I could walk outside, even at times I could run. I was starting to have more good days then bad. I really had to change everything about my life, from stress to the food that I eat to what I drink. I could no longer have a can of coke, or a slice of cake. I needed to avoid sugar, and gluten. From all the research I had been doing, I found out these things makes the Lyme worse.

The first few months giving up my favorites things were difficult, but I needed to get better. I found out when I gave up gluten after about a week I didn't have stomach pain any longer. I still have my one cup of coffee a day, but I also drink detox tea and add only stevia to it. No sugar at all. I had to learn to make meals that are healthy, mostly vegetables. At first that was very difficult, but I learned as I went.

The one big thing I had to learn it to try to get rid of the stress in my life. I had to stop talking to people that I felt were not allowing me to get well. Even if I met a negative person in my area, I would remove myself from the situation. I did not need any more stress in my life. I was fighting a huge battle every day to get well, and I needed to focus on me for once. I had spent years taking care of my kids, seeing to my husband's needs, now it was time for me to put myself first. This was difficult for me as I have always been the type of person to take care of everything. Well, I found out I can't do that anymore.

My husband and I have had our problems over the years, but I love this man. I have loved him my whole life. I wouldn't have blamed him for walking out on me. I was no longer a wife; he spent his nights helping me out of the bath or trying to make sure I didn't fall again because of the seizures. When I am too sick he goes to the store to get us food to make sure I have healthy things to eat. Throughout my treatment he did whatever he could to pay for each visit, so I didn't have to worry about where the money was coming from. I am grateful for him every day, even though at times I don't show it. I don't know what I would have done without him.

After a while the Lyme found its way around the treatment and just stopped working. I had to move on and find a different doctor. Also, I am not 100% believing that Zyto machine because I have talked to people that it showed like gallbladder issues, and they have had theirs removed. So, I do not think I would ever go that route again, but it's your personal choice to find what works for you and what doesn't.

Chapter 7: The dark side of Lyme disease: Co-infections and Parasites

When I first started treatment, I was throwing up parasites. I talked to many people with Lyme disease, and found out that so many people have these issues. I found that it's very important to kill off the parasites in our bodies. Some people can't get well without doing a parasite kill throughout their Lyme treatment. I also found that because my body did not detox well I had lots of ammonia building up in my body. I could literally smell the ammonia on my skin. The best way to rid this is to detox your body each day. You can use baths, saunas, medication. Whatever it takes. I have tried all of it. I found that drinking a spoonful of apple cider vinegar has helped with the ammonia and helps me detox. I even pour a cup in my baths now to detox my skin.

Another thing to consider is doing an organic coffee enema to rid the toxins that build up in our bodies. I feel that anyway we can get all the bad stuff out will help us start to feel better. I also make a healthy smoothie a day and add cilantro to it. I found that drinking a healthy smoothie a day, is keeping my weight down, and making me feel better. You can make all types of smoothies. I like fruit, and kale ones. All you need is a cheap blender and you are on your way to a healthier body.

Also, something that must be considered is that Lyme can be sexually transmitted. They say it's harder for a woman to pass it on to a man than vice versa, but I don't believe that. Women can also pass it on to their unborn children, as there are whole families with this disease. We need to be careful. We need to spray our families and be proactive because once you have Lyme disease you just have it, and it's very difficult to recover once it hits the chronic stage.

I found out I no longer make excuses for not feeling well. I just say I am sick and that's that. I will not try to prove to anyone that just because I look okay, I am not okay. I have seen so many doctors, have been lied to, and pushed around that I don't feel I owe anyone an explanation anymore. The only person I owe anything to is me. I need to get well, and if that means I need to take a nap every day or take up to five baths a day. I am going to do it. With this disease you must put yourself first, because if we don't we will not get better, and staying sick is not a choice for me. I want my life back.

Have you ever felt like you are trying to climb an impossibly tall mountain? It's like the more I try to find the underlying cause of what is making me sick the more mountains are being put in my path. I have worked pretty much my whole life. I was a great student, an excellent worker, now I can't remember what day of the week we are on. I have found that since I live in Illinois, most doctors do not believe we have Lyme disease and co-infections in this state. I went to have my blood drawn at a specific lab, because I had a Lyme and co-infection test I needed to get done. When I walked in I was treated very well, until the company realized that I was getting a Lyme test done, and not by someone in this state. The way I was treated after that was horrible. I do not believe that anyone should be treated in such a way by any doctors or doctor's offices. I can promise you this lab will never see me again. Yes, they were fired too.

Here are just some of the parasites I have killed throughout my almost six-year period of killing Lyme. I tested negative for parasites, but it's obvious I have them.

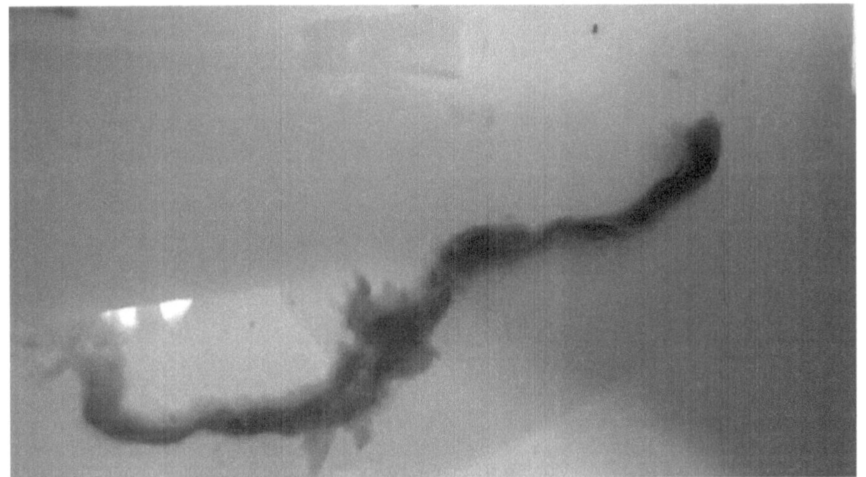

These two came out together; it was like the mother and child parasite, I have never seen anything like and it, and haven't since.

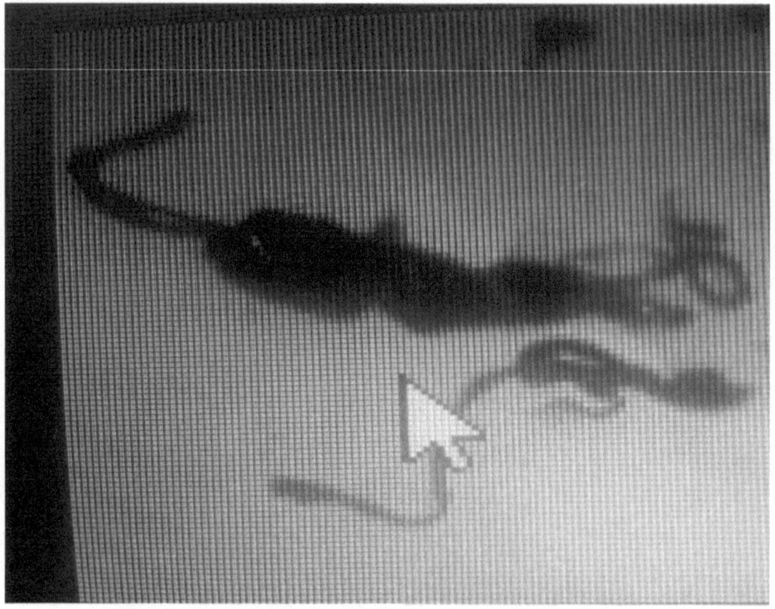

This one I was choking on, and it came out. I think it may be a possible tape worm, it has little ridges on it.

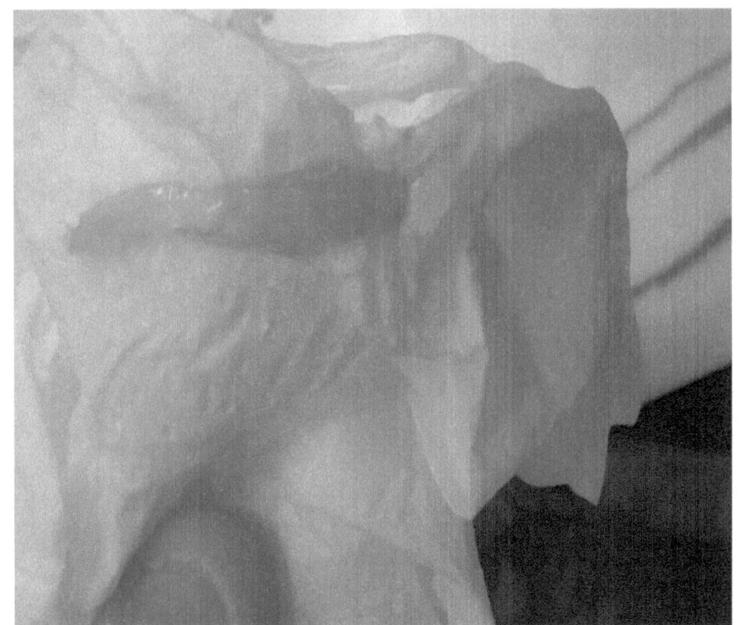

These looked like noodles, and they came in like a nest. So strange.

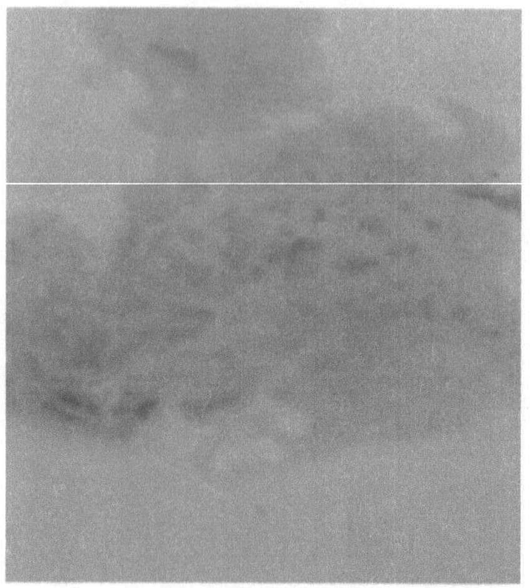

I have tried many different things to kill parasites I tried mms, goat dewormer, I would not recommend anyone of these but the para one or the off brand of it. The reason I say this is the MMS put me in the hospital with a stomach infection. What I found to work the best is a product called para one. Now, they sell the same product <u>MIMOSA PUDICA</u> on amazon for much cheaper then what I paid for the para one. It the same exact product, but just a cheaper version of it. I first saw this product on the Lyme disease summit, and I have been using it ever since. I always do a parasite kill before and after the new moon, since the parasites seem to like to reproduce around this time.

Once we start killing parasites what we must remember is that they release toxins, and we need to clear those toxins out of our bodies. What I normally do is use the parasite kill, wait three hours, and then use a binder like activated charcoal to soak up the toxins. The next day I will use some yucca root and some heapto synergy by apex separately around two hours apart and follow up with an enema to make sure I get the toxins out. To me honestly, it's a form of ammonia, or at least that is what I think it is. It smells like ammonia. I also drink an organic detox tea, that helps. It's made by Yogi and I get it from Walmart.

Chapter 8: Trying to help others, and explain this disease

I spend most of my day trying to research ways to help me, and other people like me. Some days I am just too sick to get out of bed, so I just write things in my notebook, hoping to research them later. In truth if you have Lyme disease or a co-infection of Lyme, you probably already have had people in your life not believe you, maybe even think you need mental help. It's very difficult for a person that is well to understand that one minute I could be fine, and the next my body freezes up, and I can't take one step. That physically I look normal but inside my body is burning like I am being electrocuted, and it could happen at any time of the day or night. I don't ask for people to really understand, but that they just try to have compassion. Before I was sick I finished my Law classes with a 4.0 grade point average. Now I can't remember simple words or terms.

Throughout this sickness, I have lost many things. At first the seizures just cost me my job, then my ability to drive, then my ability to walk. Finally, I found that because I wasn't a typical sick person, some people just preferred to ignore I exist. Maybe that is why I felt I needed to help as many people as I can, by reaching out to them online. I can give them information on Lyme literature doctors, and treatment plans that I am using in hopes that it will help them too. When I am well enough I research as much as I possibly can, because I feel with this disease we must be our own doctors, advocates, and supporters.

At first because there was so much stigma with Lyme I would tell people I had something else; I had Autoimmune disease or even MS. It was almost like I had to hide the disease I really had to get people to understand why I was always sick. Then one day I just realized why I am hiding the truth? Why am I lying? I stopped trying to explain to people that Lyme isn't cured with three weeks of medicine for some people a whole lot of people exactly. The top Lyme doctor in New York said there is about a twenty-day window, and then you go chronic. I was treated a little over a month after getting sick, but I am not sure how long I really had Lyme. I mean looking about over my life I had health issues even as a child. My mother told me they thought I had leukemia when I was a baby. I was in the hospital quite a bit she once told me. As the years started to go by soon everyone knew or now knows someone with Lyme. My experience with Lyme was so bad, that I don't want others to suffer like I did. I doubted myself so many times I even thought maybe I was crazy. It took me talking to so many others going through the exact same thing for me to realize we all have this chronic disease. We are fighting for our lives.

Now with Lyme we have online support groups where we can go on, ask questions as some people on these sites are medical professionals, but that have Lyme themselves and can't get better. Some have reached remission. We in these groups try our best to not judge other people. We just try to be helpful. If someone is having a really hard time, we all try and give them support and let them know they are not alone. In 2012 when I first became sick, I didn't know anyone that had Lyme. I didn't know anyone that could walk one day and be in a wheelchair the next. I felt my life was over, but what I didn't realize is that I was going to get a new life. I feel that Lyme Disease has taught me to have compassion in a way that I probably didn't have before. It has taught me that life is very precious, and that each day that we wake up, no matter how much pain we are in, is still a good day.

In 2017 a Lyme friend of mine passed away. She had been trying to help me, we were around the same age. She died at age forty, I am forty-two now. When the Lyme community lost her, we lost a great person, a great friend. I took her death very hard, and I realized that no matter what happens I will not let the world forget her. She died because she couldn't get proper treatment in Iowa. I almost didn't make it because I couldn't get proper treatment in Illinois. Our stories are very similar. She is not the first death in the Lyme community, there have been many, many deaths. Some died in their sleep, some killed themselves because they couldn't get help.

This is not acceptable. No one should have to die because they can't get treatment. I am sorry, but the government should not tell us how to treat our disease. There is scientific data showing that Lyme is still detectable in mice that were treated with antibiotics. https://www.niaid.nih.gov/diseases-conditions/lyme-disease-antibiotic-treatment-research

This study was done in 2008, It's 2018 and we are still being told three weeks of antibiotics is going to cure all of us. That is complete bullshit.

There has been testing done in Germany that showed Lyme in mosquitoes. These kinds of tests have never been done here in the United States that I am aware of. https://www.ncbi.nlm.nih.gov/pubmed/26631488 I still believe that people are getting Lyme here from mosquitoes, spiders, and I know of a lady in Michigan that became infected with Lyme from a horsefly. To me if it bites, it can transmit.

I spend so much of my time telling people to spray their families, and make sure their pets are protected. Once you have Lyme, it's already too late for me to tell you how to protect yourself. I saw an article the other day where this lady had two inside cats and was out in her garden. Later, she found ticks on her cats. We must be very careful now, these bugs are just about everywhere, and I know that the mosquitoes are horrible this year.

Chapter 9: When you realize you are not well enough to work

I always thought the next doctor will fix me; the next medicine will be my cure. Recently I realize there isn't a real cure. Three weeks of doxy did not cure me, and thousands of dollars on self-treatment did not cure me either. I had to change my way of thinking just like I had to change my diet. I believe the only way to have a semi normal life with this disease is to find a Lyme doctor, and a damn good one. I needed to find one that could help me with my seizures, that proved to me impossible here in Illinois. I also came to realize that I since we couldn't get the seizures to stop I wouldn't be able to go back into my accounting career that I loved.

I kept putting off applying for disability, because I felt like I was kind of giving in to this illness. It was like the day I had to sale my car because I could no longer drive it. I felt like my heart was breaking into tiny pieces, and there wasn't anything I could really do about it. I must have went on the disability website 100 times. Each time talking myself out of applying. I valued myself for my ability to make money, my ability to do a great job, and help my husband provide for my family. Lyme disease took all of that away from me. It stripped my self-esteem, with each doctor telling me I had something else, pushing me to another doctor, other diagnoses, and I lost myself somewhere. I often felt if I could not support my family, what good was I in this life?

We can't allow this disease to take over our minds this way. We may never have a normal life because of this disease, but really what is considered normal? I have bad days, I have seizures, so yes, some days I can't walk very well, but the days that I can, I feel like I can accomplish anything. The good days are very rare, so we must have cherished them. I think I finally had to make the disability decision when life kind of made it for me.

I applied for disability. I was denied and had to fight for three years to win. My disability paperwork says chronic Lyme on it, because my doctor still feels this is what's wrong with me, even though at the time we were told there was no Lyme here in Illinois. To this day she is still my primary doctor because she believed me when no one else did.

I have been working since I was sixteen years old, the only time I did not work was when my daughter was little. I took care of her at home until she was almost two years old. Going from having a job and making my own money to not making anything was very hard for me. I don't ask people for anything. I even have a hard time asking my husband for things. I am the kind of person that feels if I can't buy it myself I don't need it. For three years I did not have an income, so I had to get over this somewhat. I am still a very proud person, but I am also a logical person, and I needed to survive. For me to do that, I needed to treat my disease. This takes money, and quite a bit of it.

It's hard for me to answer when people ask me what I do, or what's my job. I used to have a career, and now I am just a mom and a wife. Some days I am an advocate, and some days I am just trying to still survive this day, this week. If you're taking the time to read this book you should know I am not a professional writer, my daughter is bringing my story to life for me. I just needed to tell my story so that maybe it can help someone else. I bet there are so many people just like me that just became sick, in fact I know there is.

For me disability was a hard choice. I still would prefer to work. The only issue is my body is not allowing me to do that yet. I still have seizures. Yes, six years almost of seizures. I do better when I am busy. When I am working and making my own money. I had a very difficult time staying at home all the time. I think one of the hardest things for me is that I don't have the energy to even keep my whole house clean to this day. I find that even if I must fold laundry it can sometimes take me hours to do just one load. My energy, once it gets depleted, that's it. I can't seem to recharge.

When I am not trying to figure out how to calm my symptoms or help someone else with Lyme I still love music of all kinds. It has really helped me through some rough things in my life. I think we all must find things that make us happy, no matter what that is. For me I love flowers, animals, children, and music. So anytime I am having a really bad day my animals seem to sense it. I have three cats and an older dog. They are my babies. They follow me around and if I have a seizure the dog and eldest cat will stand at my head waiting for me to come out of it.

Chapter 10: Going Backwards

I realized I was getting worse, and not better. The NP , I was seeing was trying everything, but I wasn't getting better anymore. The seizures were more intense, and the pain was out of control. I spoke to her, and she realized she couldn't help me much longer. I honestly am not sure if the doctors in Illinois know enough about Lyme to really help me. She did tell me about another doctor, one that she thought could help me with the seizures, I had my appointment in November. I talked to many of this doctor's patients, and he is really helping them get better. My case is a little bit difficult because of the mold, Lyme, and seizures, but I feel I need to try him.

The thing is most Lyme doctors are out of state and most of these doctors can't take insurance for fear that if they continue to treat a person with Lyme long term the insurance companies will shut them down. This has happened over and over in other states, so doctors are scared to treat Lyme patients. The out of pocket cost for treatment is very expensive. I know for myself personally; I have spent thousands of dollars on medicine that has not helped me and have spent so much money on treatment that just didn't work. When you are so sick, you become so desperate that you are almost willing to try anything. Mostly everyone in Illinois must go out of state for this treatment.

As I have had lots of time to think, I had to realize my body is in bad shape because of a lot of things. I worked in a manufacturing company for years. I was exposed to many different chemicals. I was living in a house that was filled with black mold, and I was under an intense amount of stress because the job I loved was moving to another part of the country. I do believe all these factors helped me get this sick. I do not believe the mosquito or bug alone did this to my body. I do believe in the saying that our body is like an onion with many different layers. We must treat all the layers of the body when we are this ill. We need to change our eating habits, we need to detox our bodies, and find a way to relieve some stress in our life.

Some days when I can't get out of bed, I just cry. I cry because I feel like I have lost so much, and I cry because I want to walk, work, drive, and I can't. I look out the window and see everyone coming and going living their life, and I ask myself how did I get here? I often ask myself were there signs that I had ignored. Of course, there were, I was so busy working, and living my life, I didn't realize how sick I was becoming. I think it really took me having to fall on the floor time, and time again for me to realize I can't worry about the fact I am not well enough to cook, I can't go grocery shopping, or go to a movie. I had to focus on getting well and being happy with the things I can do.

On August 19th, I woke up like every day; in pain, with stiff legs, but today I felt a little worse. My body was aching, and I felt like I had some type of flu. This is normal for Lyme patients, so I didn't think too much about it. I was trying to make it to the bathroom when a seizure hit. I couldn't stop the shaking, my whole body gave into it, and I found myself falling. I remember hitting my head on the ceramic tile, and that was the last thing I recall. When I came to my husband was there and he helped me to the car and to the nearest hospital. In the emergency room, the seizures took over again, and they rushed me into a room right away. The doctor saw me, and for once in a whole year, he didn't look at me like I faked these seizures. He diagnosed me with a seizure disorder, gave me medication to try to stop them, and sent me home.

The seizure medication helps but does not stop or control the seizures. I also have been taking Gaba pills to help with them when I feel them coming on. I have researched so much over the past year trying to figure out what is wrong with me. I often feel I know more about some of these viruses and diseases then doctors do. I feel that with Lyme or with any disease, the patient must be their own advocate, we owe it to our bodies to be informed.

After that day, I realized I can't control these seizures anymore, and if I can't get a doctor to cure me, I am going to have to start getting them to try to treat me per symptom. Most doctors in Illinois did not believe we had Lyme disease here, and especially since my second Lyme test was negative they figured I cured myself or had some other autoimmune disorder. Most doctors were not aware that Lyme disease is usually followed by different co-infections. When the tick bites us, or mosquito, or whatever, it has other viruses in them that we are infected with. So, since most doctor are looking for Lyme disease in a test that is not accurate, they assume we are not sick, or it's something else. At that point they are just leaving us to get worse, or in some cases die.

I am not about to give up like that. I had to fight my whole life. I grew up poor, and I had to fight for everything I had. I always thought I would be at a different place in my life then to be 37 on a cane, without a job, and begging a doctor to help me. I have a different attitude when I go into a doctor's office now. I may not be a doctor, but I have researched Lyme disease, and all the co-infections for a year. A year where twenty plus doctors either refused to help me or could not. I laid in bed, too sick to get out, in too much pain, crying just to use the washroom, so I have had plenty of time to think about this disease in a whole new light. When I walk in a doctor's office, I start out by saying I was positive for Lyme in 2012, and I continue to get worse, do you think you can help me or not?

In September almost, a year to the date of being diagnosed, I started looking around for another doctor. My case is not as cut and dry as some of the other Lyme patients. I get horrible seizures, I have mold issues, and my body was being poisoned where I was working. The pain has gotten so bad, that I started taking prescription painkillers, they didn't help a whole lot, so my sister started to research, and found me some nettle leaf that works pretty good for the pain.

Chapter 11: Pain

I wanted to talk about Lyme pain here. When the seizures come on, it feels like I am being shocked from the inside out. My whole-body jerks and moves in abnormal ways that I can't control. I am conscious of what is going on around me, but I can't do anything to stop it. My husband tries everything in his power to help me, but most of the time, he just can hold me while I cry. I had two children, and I can tell you by far Lyme pain is the worst pain I have ever felt in my life.

I have tried different painkillers; Norco, tramadol, naproxen, but I found the nettle leaf to work the best for me so far. My sister buys it by the bottles, so I have it when I need it, and I really appreciate that because without a job money is tight. We do the best we can, but my treatment has taken every extra penny we have had, and so much we didn't have.

For pain I have made ginger tea. I buy fresh whole ginger, cut up a piece, and boiling it in water with honey and lemon. I also use turmeric for inflammation, both helps some, but when it gets too bad the only real relief I get it taking a bath so hot it almost burns my skin. I feel like we must do whatever it takes to get us out of this pain, the pain itself will make a person crazy.

Even without the seizures my arms, and legs feel like they are on fire. Sometimes they tingle, but most of the time they just burn. They even turn red, and so does my face when it gets bad. I get a weird pressure in my head, sometimes it feels like water is overflowing in my brain. My eyes tend to go blurry, and I lose my focus all the time. I tell myself this is temporary, and it will pass, but I am not sure how long it will take for everything to back to normal.

I am fighting this disease with everything I have, I look to God to help me, to guide me, but inside I know I must be strong enough to beat this. This isn't something anyone can do for me, I must find the strength to keep fighting when I am in so much pain, I want to give up, I want to give in. I wish my mother was still alive. I know that she would help me, she would comfort me, but I feel she is help guiding me from heaven. There are bad days when I think I can't take anymore, and I always see a little light at the end of the tunnel. I always feel like it could get worse, so let's give it a little more fight.

It had come to the point where nettle isn't working any longer, and I had to investigate pain medicine. I tried tramadol, and it really didn't do that much for me. I honestly believe that I had to get the inflammation levels down before the pain went down. I am a firm believer in cbd products and feel anyone with Lyme should investigate them. Your pain medicine is your own personal choice, just know that if your pain is to high it will affect your immune system. At least I found this to be true for me.

Chapter 12: Not wanting to explain why you're not well

The last few months, I have been stuck in one room. I don't get outside much, even to just sit in my chair. I am mostly in bed as my legs just don't work the way they should. It almost gets to a point that I just don't want to explain it to people anymore. Yes, sometimes I can walk, and other days I must use a cane. For some reason people don't seem to understand that, they think oh you have Lyme disease take two weeks or three weeks of antibiotics, and you're cured. I wish it was that simple, because if it was we would all be cured. I have had people try to suggest I made myself this way.

My response is this: I can no longer drive, I can't go into a store, and walk around half the time. I can't cook for myself, because I can't make it down the stairs. There are days I just skip eating because I can't make it downstairs, and I'm just too sick to eat. Or my kids or husband must get me something to eat. I would love to go for a walk and use my legs to walk, not far, maybe a block or two. I can't do that anymore. I would love to go to a job, where I was needed, a job that I could do. Before Lyme disease, I had all of this. I think most importantly I would love to not have to have my son have to lay in bed with me to play cards, because I am too sick to get out of bed. Or have both my kids had to sit with me because they both know I can't get downstairs or go anywhere. I would love to take them places to have fun again to be a mom again. I miss it so very much.

So, when a doctor or a person says to me well you don't look sick, I must really hold back on what I want to say. I really want to say, "Well, you don't look stupid either, but it quite obvious you are.". Would someone tell a cancer patient they don't look sick enough? No, they would not, so I don't know why people feel like because we have Lyme disease they can say whatever they want? Do I sound a little pissed off? I think we need to find our anger with this disease, it will help us get through the really bad time, and believe me, there are going to be some really difficult times.

We are now in November 2013, I have been in bed about two months now. It's been months since I have been to a grocery store, or out shopping. My legs do not work, my seizures are bad, I haven't found a medicine that has completely stopped them. I continue to research as much as I can, I feel like at times I am an animal trapped in a cage, only the cage is my body. I tell it to move, it doesn't. My brain tells my legs to move, they don't. So, I am trapped.

I used to be such a proud person, so stubborn, and had to do everything myself. I have found with this disease, I could no longer do simple tasks. On Monday, I was having intense pain, only a hot bath would help. My husband helps me to the bathroom and gets the bath ready. I couldn't even pour the epsom salt into the bath, because my hands were not working right. I started to soak in the bathroom, and I go into a full-blown seizure. I wanted to call out for help, but I can't find my voice. Lucky for me my hands were jerking so much my wedding band was hitting the side of the tub. I was sinking under the water, and I couldn't pull myself up. My husband rushed in to save me, and I realized in a lot of ways he has been saving me lately. Every time I feel like I can't do this anymore he is there to say, "We will find something to help you, we will keep searching.".

What I had to realize, and I think anyone dealing with a chronic illness must come to terms with, it's this disease, is not my fault. I am not lazy. I am sick. If I need to take two naps a day or five baths just to live a somewhat normal life, then so be it. Also, if the pain gets so bad, and it will get so bad with Lyme, that you want to die, because you can't take it any longer, I feel you do whatever it takes for you to feel better. To me that means if you must take herbs, narcotics, you must do what is best for you. I feel like I know my body, I know how much pain I can take, and how much I can't.

Let's talks about the mental side of this disease. Do I feel depressed? Hell, yes, I do. I want to do so many things that I can't. I don't want my children to have to take care of me. I should be taking care of them. This disease will get in your head and convince you that you would be better off dead than alive. When thoughts like this happen to me, I tell myself, it's the Lyme disease trying to get you, you are strong, you are brave, you can do it. I also think about my kids, my family, my husband, I haven't come this far to give up. I am not allowing the Lyme to win, and that is just what it's trying to do. It's trying to beat me.

In 2016 , Illinois made medical cannabis legal for people with certain medical issues and seizures. We came up with the money I applied and was approved. I found that they had patches that helped with my pain. Now if you're against this, that is your own personal choice, but for me, it has saved me more times than I can count. I was on pain pills, but I found them to not work very well. Or I would have to keep taking more and I didn't want to do that. Some of the side effects were also bad.

If you can get a hold of some cbd oil, in most cases if you're not allergic to it should help some. I won't say it takes away all the Lyme pain because if your symptoms are flaring sometimes only time will help ease up the pain. If you experience this, please know you don't owe anything to anyone, you don't need to explain yourself. I only say this because for a long time I apologized for being sick. I am not sure why I did this, but I felt bad because I was too sick to do much of anything. I no longer apologize, and neither should you. A person with cancer doesn't have to say they are sorry, and I refused to for Lyme. I talk about cancer a lot and I know I compare the disease. I do this because I had a family member go through cancer, and I feel both diseases will try and take your life.

Chapter 13: New Doctor, New Hope

 For the last three months I have been stuck in bed, when I stand I get dizzy and fall. I now can do a bare minimum, I need help with basics things like getting to the bathroom or to take a bath. I can no longer cook for myself or my family, so most of my meals are spent sitting up in bed. I am too weak to make it down the stairs anymore. On my online support group some of the ladies have told me about a new doctor. He knows quite a bit about mold illness, and may be able to help me, as he handles difficult cases. I set up an appointment with him, the first visit is expensive at 475.00 I knew it would take some time to come up with the money. My first visit was set for November 25th, 2013.

I was nervous about seeing another doctor. Would he think I was crazy? Would he try to diagnose me with some other weird disease that we both know I did not have? On the first visit, I had my list of symptoms ready, a timeline of my health issues printed out, along with all tests I have had done. I wanted to have everything ready because in the past I have gotten confused and forgotten what I was supposed to say. The ladies on the online support group had helped me with this and called me a few weeks before the appointment to make sure I knew what I needed to get the most out of the appointment. I could tell right from the beginning this doctor was extremely smart.

I had taken a mold test before going into his office, and failed it horribly, not surprising since the old house we had to move out of was covered in mold. He really listened to what I had to say and went over everything with me. He didn't make me feel crazy, and I felt comfortable with him. He drew up a lab report and sent me in for 17 blood tests. The testing center told me since some of the tests had to go far out, it would take a few weeks for my results to come back. About two weeks later I received an email from the doctor going over some of the tests. I tested positive for mycoplasma, I have chemical poisoning, and my body is toxic. For once in over a year, we had some answers. He had known what to look for in my blood and found it. I had a few other Lyme co-infections, and would start medication right away.

I started on CSM right away, it's a binder, and removed toxins from our bodies. I have been exposed to so much mold and toxins from the places I have worked that my body was in rough shape. I had found out I have the gene that does not allow me to detox, so in the past when I was getting antibiotics I had become worse instead of better. On the Cholestyramine I became worse instead of better at first, it gave me a four-day headache. In a few weeks I started to see a little improvement, things like pain eased up some, and my seizures which were out of control with 4 packs of medication were easing up some on a lower dose.

It has now been four months with me being stuck in bed. Four months where I no longer have a life. My legs just stopped working for me, my body freezes up, and I fall. I am having ear pain, burning feet, burning hands, to the point that I just cry.

Now some people say prescription painkillers are bad for us, I say if you are in this type of pain, take what you need to feel better. If we had another disease besides Lyme people wouldn't be so fast to judge us. For some reason because its Lyme, and not too many people understand the disease, they think they can tell us what is right for our bodies. I say before you judge, put yourself in that person's shoes.

It seems almost weekly we are now reading where Lyme warriors are dying, this saddens me to the core. Not only are they dying because the disease has not been treated, the health care has failed them because they can't take it anymore and decide to end it. The pain is so bad at times, it takes my breath away. I am a person that understands how some of the Lyme people may think that suicide is the answer, but what they don't realize is no matter how bad it is, it's only temporary, you can have five bad days and one good day. You just must keep fighting, keep going. I was in the same spot as them, a few months back, if it wasn't for someone reaching out to me, I am not sure what would have happened. Now I just feel like I haven't fought this much for nothing. I didn't go through forty-five plus doctors, told I was crazy, to just give up now. I am ready to fight. I want my life back, I don't want to be afraid to go outside. It shouldn't worry me all the time if what if I seize, what if I fall?

I think when you get infected with something like Lyme, or really any disease, it changes you. At this point I have been sick over a year, a year without answers but more questions. Finally, when my tests results came back, it was like the pieces of the puzzle were fitting together. For the first time in a long time, I no longer feel that I must prove to anyone that I am sick. If I can't do something I just say I can't do it and move on, I am not going to feel bad about it, no one should. I often wonder what happens if I do not get better? From most of the research that I have done late stage Lyme is not curable, the only thing I can hope for is remission. What happens if one day I decide I can't do this anymore? It's at these times when I think about my kids, my husband, my animals, my friends, my Lyme friends, and my family. If I give up I hurt them, and I don't want to hurt them anymore than this disease has already.

The reality is holidays are going to come and go, and we are not going to be able to attend. The simplest things like, putting up a tree is now impossible for me to do. My ten-year-old son put the tree up, my kids had to get it from the basement, as I couldn't make it down there. I found myself unable to make dinner, unable to celebrate, like we normally did. The holidays made me sad, because it just showed me all the things I couldn't do, all the things I was missing. My kids now understand that I lay down more than I am up, certain things I can no longer do, they realize what Lyme does to a person, how it destroys a person's life.

I can say I have pulled away from people. I find that when I am home away from everyone I feel safer. Since I don't know when I will seize up, just the thought of it will stress me out, and I don't want other people to stare at me. I try to explain what Lyme pain feels like, but most of the time I can't put it into words. I feel like I can't be the person I once was, I am not even sure who I am anymore. I am now on a strict diet, food no longer brings me pleasure. Everything that I once thought was important has changed for me. I worry that my kids see me sick, see me weak. It's hard for me to understand this disease; imagine how it is for a child.

It's cold and snowing here in Illinois, and the cold hurts my legs to the bone. I can't go outside, not even for short periods without feeling intense pain. While this new doctor is good, I couldn't afford to keep seeing him at 475 a visit plus medicine. Also, he moved to another state anyway. Insurance wouldn't even cover my medicine: they were charging me five dollars a pill. I didn't even have an income, how was I going to pay for that. In 2013 and 2014 those were the roughest years for me, I was fighting for disability and fighting to live. I felt like my husband was getting sick of me being sick, I mean how much can a person take? He would go to work I would be in bed. He would come home I would still be in bed. I needed assistance just getting to the bathroom at times, every part of my body would stop working.

I think the worst day was at one point, he had brought me a salad. I was in my wheelchair, as I could no longer walk, and I tried to eat the salad. My brain would not tell my hand where to put the salad, and everything fell on the floor. I remember just sitting there crying. He had to walk away from me for a minute because it really upset him to see me like this. I now had like ALS symptoms, and I even had a neurologist tell me I may have it or MS. It wasn't that, it was Lyme for me all along. Honestly, I believe if you or your loved one have been diagnosed with either disease, send your blood to Germany and let them look for tick borne diseases. The company is called Armin Labs, it could save a life.

I had to drop out of school because I could no longer follow or do the homework. I had a bad seizure and it caused some brain damage on the left side on my brain.

Yes, those 'fake' seizures caused me to get brain damage. When I think back about how I was treated, how we all are treated with Lyme it makes me very angry. I mean who do these doctor's think they are? What happened to their oath to treat the patient?

Around this time, I started seeing a new primary doctor because I lost my good insurance and had to see a state doctor. Let me tell you she was a work of art that one. She constantly told me to lose weight. To get down on the floor and do yoga when I couldn't even get on the floor at that time. When I would shake and seize, she took my husband to another room and told him I had PTSD and could stop the seizures if I really wanted to. Imagine a doctor telling your loved one, the person that is taking care of you, that you are faking this illness. That if you just wanted it bad enough you could get better, you could be better. I would like to say that my husband believed me, but I think of hearing it from a doctor, at first, he kind of believed her. I started to hide my symptoms, I didn't want to be a burden to anyone.

I will be honest with you all reading this. I told my husband to find someone else, to just divorce me, and find someone well. I couldn't guarantee him that I would ever be well again. I just didn't know. I was doing everything I could, but I was still having about 20 seizures a day. I tried everything I could; seizures medicine, gluten free, Lyrica, gabapentin, nothing worked for me. I started to think that the seizures have to be caused by the infection, either the toxins, or the parasites associated with the Lyme. I knew I had parasites, I saw them, even though the parasite test was negative. I later found out the parasite tests had to be done at a special place and around a certain time of month to really get a positive test. I stopped trying to convince people I was sick, I just started working on getting better.

It had become so bad that in Elmwood Park I could hear the 90 cta stop all the way outside. The sound seemed like it had been amplified 1000 times. I literally had to wear ear plugs to be able to lay in bed. I would shake and cry. I even had to black out the light in my room, the sound and light hurt me so much I just couldn't handle it. Around this time, I thought I would be better off dead than alive. I felt trapped in my body, a burden to my family. The pain was so bad that I considered cutting my own legs off. I know that sounds crazy, but the Lyme was making me crazy. I was hallucinating, my brain felt like it was on fire, and I would think that I saw spiders or bugs everywhere. At one point I argued with my husband to give me my roller skates, and I hadn't been skating since I was like eight years old. Then, I was convinced he had taken my car keys and hid my car. The sad thing was I didn't even remember selling my car, and I hadn't drove in years at this point.

Chapter 14: Change is coming/Mercury removal

It is now 2018, things are starting to change, new articles are coming out about Lyme now. The television is even talking about Lyme now. In both Lyme groups that I am in, the numbers of members keep growing. In every state Lyme is getting so out of hand, so many people are getting infected. It's not just the Lyme either, it's other tick-borne diseases. I saw a news report where a 2-year-old died from a tick bite in Indiana. These diseases and bugs are killing people.

May 16th, 2018

Today I woke up nervous, there is a Lyme bill in the Senate that is waiting for a vote. This Lyme bill was named after a little girl here in Illinois that became sick and could not get treatment. Her and her mother and some other Lyme patients went down to Springfield and told their stories. Starting in 2012 I had reached out to the president at the time, senators, etc., but because at that time there was not enough people in Illinois with Lyme people didn't listen to me. This year I started to get emails back, one was from an email I sent in 2016. It was from our senator here in the DuPage office. They were interested in what happened to me and started to ask me questions. Also, this year the paper ran my story about not being able to get treatment here in Illinois. My part in trying to help others get this bill passed. I just reached out to senators and reps, I told them my story, and how I can't get treatment here. I spent as much time as I could be reaching out to them, and sometimes when I was able to I made phone calls.

This bill would allow doctors in Illinois to treat us. The people that were left behind. The people that were sick, and abandoned, and who were left to our own devices. In the past doctors have told me here they can't treat me, I have had my three weeks of oral antibiotics, and they can't risk treating me anymore. This bill protects the doctor's and allows them to treat a Lyme patient how they see fit. People just don't understand how we can be sick, and only allowed three weeks of treatment.

The bill passed 56 to zero, and its making its way to the governor office. I was crying like a baby. Until a person is so sick with a disease that they feel like they are going to die, and not able to get treatment they will not understand how bad Lyme is. We have literally spent every penny we had trying to keep my symptoms at bay, so I can be somewhat functional. I no longer need the wheelchair, but some days I still get the seizures, and get so dizzy I can barely make it to the bathroom. The pain gets so bad still that on these days I cry because I can't get relief.
For me getting better has been very slow, and sometimes I feel like I take two steps forward and three steps back. If I have a lot of stress I go backwards, and sometimes we can't avoid stress. I am starting to have more good days then bad now. I am starting to cook more, laugh more, and sometimes I even find myself dancing a little. Maybe I am just happy to be alive or maybe I am just happy to have a day where I am not having seizures, or my pain is more manageable.

Mercury removal

On December 11th, 2017 I had the remaining three mercury filled teeth removed. I went to a biomedical dentist in Downers Grove. At first, I was really scared to get it done. I had done my research and found that it was dangerous to take them out. If it was not done properly a person could reabsorbed the mercury. I had talked in length about the procedure, and this office used a smart system; they used charcoal, oxygen, and even a dam that went into my mouth, so I didn't swallow any mercury. I was suited up, and they were suited up. I felt some pulling, and tugging, but nothing painful. It was over quickly. Less than two hours. The dentist office redid my x-rays to make sure all the mercury was out, and it was.

Afterwards I had a slight headache, a sore jar, then a little nausea. I kind of felt like I had a slight flu, but from reading the material the books that were giving to me prior to the procedure I found out this was normal. After one night of it, I am feeling back to normal the next day. I never realized that teeth could make you sick. Well, after doing some research I realized that teeth can hold in bacteria, infections and, yes, even Lyme. In the past I had a metal filling removed without the dentist taking special precautions. I was literally sick for two months afterwards.

If you have metal fillings in your mouth my suggestion is to have a biomedical dentist look your case over for you. Over time the metal will start to leak into your mouth and even your blood stream. This can cause anything from autoimmune diseases to mood disorders and pain. The dentists don't tell you this when they put this stuff in your mouth. I never thought that I had to worry about my teeth, but after I became sick with Lyme and I could not get better I had to look at everything that was going on with my body. I had constant tooth pain when I had the mercury in my mouth, I did not realize that my teeth were helping me stay sick. This goes back to the onion theory. It's not one thing making us sick, but layers of things, and we must get through all the layers to get well.

Chapter 15: Getting out of the wheelchair

People ask me how I got out of the wheelchair, and I will be honest. I never stopped trying to figure this out. I killed parasites, I detox the ammonia out of my body, I used to tell doctors I smell ammonia and they looked at me like I was nuts. What I figured out is as I kill this stuff off, my body gets flooded with ammonia. I can't detox it, so I had to do things like coffee enemas, take a medicine called L methionine, another medicine called hepato synergy that opens my pathways, and others. I have been researching things like LDN, or Low dose Naltrexone because I knew my immune system was in bad shape. I like what I read about this drug and asked doctors to put me on it, many did not. I found a doctor here in Schaumburg who did, and it made a big difference with my pain levels. I am always researching new protocols. My theory is that this is why so many people with Lyme get ALS like symptoms. Also, why so many of us with Lyme have high liver enzymes. I know for myself my liver was so bad at one time, it was at the level of an alcoholic.

I am not embarrassed to say I have literally tried everything I could afford to, even bee venom. For me it did not work, but it has helped some others. I am desperate to get my life back. I reach out to people all the time: if they were in remission I want to know how they did it. On my bad days, I will watch a comedy or listen to music and I will allow myself to just rest. I try my best to help others with Lyme and have met so many great people doing so. I can't name everyone here, but you know who you are. I watch the Lyme summits and I take notes. I will do whatever it takes to get better.

I have had some really bad experience with doctors, but I have also had some that have tried to help me. I found a Np in Romeoville that was willing to help me, she does not treat Lyme, but does look at the whole body. She looks at things like your cd57, your inflammation levels, your vitamin levels, are you absorbing nutrients etc. With her help and with my own research I have improved myself about 50 to 60 percent on some days. Other days I am still trying to beat this disease. I use things like high dose fish oil, at least 6 grams a day to lower my inflammation levels. My liver was in such bad shape because I was killing some of the Lyme off, but it was dumping the toxins right back into my body.

I now listen to my body. I detox as much as I can. I use epsom salt baths, yucca root, detox tea, activated charcoal. When my brain feels like it's on fire, I wrap my head in a heating pad, it helps. I found a product called antitiox 11 cns /pns by jergians. It detoxes the ammonia out of the brain, this stuff works well. I use para one, which I learned about from the Lyme summits to kill parasites. I have this issue when my potassium drops, so I take potassium, otherwise I get chest pains. Some days it seems like it's a constant battle between me and the Lyme, but I am starting to win the battle because I am no longer confined to a wheelchair, or walker.

I tend to avoid hospitals, but if I must go I say I have a history of Lyme disease, and leave it at that. Some doctors will ask me how and where I became sick. I say Melrose Park. They always look a little confused, I am sorry that I didn't get my disease is some forest, but I was infected in my own backyard. Now we honestly do not know if I had Lyme my whole life and that mosquito brought it out, or what. I grew up partly in West Virginia which is known for having a ton of Lyme Disease. Now Illinois and Wisconsin are known for the same thing, so I may never know how, or which bite did this to me. My parents picked ticks off us all the time when we were little, so who really knows. I just know I have Lyme. I didn't know prior to 2012 that a bug could destroy a person's life, but it can, and it will. It will try and take everything you care about away from you, but I am not the type of person to not fight back. I read something the other day. It said it's not how many times you fall in life that matters, but how many times you get back up. If you have Lyme or any other chronic disease, you will learn what you are made of.

I have been fighting for change since I have been sick. I have emailed our passed president to our current one. I have reached out to so many senators, papers, etc. My whole goal now is to make sure no one else must go through what I did. A person shouldn't have to beg a doctor to help them only to be treated like they were either crazy or lazy. There should be laws in place to take care of doctors that want and knows how to treat a Lyme patient. The main thing that I am fighting for is that all of us with Lyme have access to treatment, here is a little bit of what was written in a news article from me. "There are so many people like me here in Illinois that suffer from a persistent Lyme infection that can't get treatment; this Lyme bill will literally save so many lives-many of which are children," said Tera of DuPage. "With Lyme and other tick-borne diseases on the rise, it's very important that we have access to affordable and adequate treatment options.

I am not going to go away or back down. I literally have reached out to people until some started to listen to me. I explained to our senators that my case is in no way unique. I could be one of their own family members. I literally went from working to a wheelchair in a very short time, and not one doctor could or would help me here, their hands were tied because I had my three weeks of treatment that at the time in 2012 were the guidelines for Lyme. I should be cured I heard over and over. Well, I wasn't, I was sick, and I am tired of being sick. No person could or would make this up. What do I get out of being this way? I lost my job, my house, my ability to drive, my ability to walk, and some days I can't even speak. I used to be a very social person, and when I became sick with Lyme I couldn't even make it down four stairs. I couldn't be around people the noise was so amplified it would literally hurt my ears. I because paranoid, anxious, and depressed. It became so bad I literally could not leave my apartment for weeks or months at a time.

I have read on the history of Lyme, I do believe this is not the same Lyme disease that infected people in the 70's or early 80's. I believe this disease had been manufactured to disable people, the disease itself morphs so that treatment and a cure is very difficult. Why do I believe this? I have literally been trying for almost six years to get better, and I realized that Lyme is a political disease. If I had cancer a doctor would help me, but since I have Lyme I can't get help, people expect us to do what, go away and die. I am sorry that is not going to happen to me, I am going to fight, and I am going to tell you what I went through in the hopes that you or your family do not have to go through this.

Chapter 16: The Herxheimer reaction

I compare Lyme to Cancer a lot in my life, because when you treat cancer what happens? You get sicker, right? The same thing happens when you treat Lyme. Both disease will attack and shut down your immune system. Both disease will make you bedridden, you will be in intense pain, throwing up, and wondering if you will ever get your life back. The only difference is if I had cancer I would have three or four doctors in my corner trying to help me. With Lyme I was left on my own to try and figure this out. I have some family that have stuck by me, but they couldn't save me. No one could. I had to learn to save myself. I will be completely blunt here, when I am killing off the Lyme lots of times I have thought to myself it would be easier to just step in front of a train or take some pills and go to sleep.

The Lyme itself is very painful, but when I start to kill it, it brings the pain and symptoms to a whole new level of hell. I can only compare it to my body being set on fire, because that is what this feels like. Now some doctors are saying to not allow the body to herx to experience the die off, and some are saying we must go through the die off to get better. It feels like my body is on fire and at the same time, someone is stabbing me with an ice pick in my brain and hitting my legs with a hammer. I have tried different things throughout these past five, almost six years to lower the effect of the herx. I have used things like Alka seltzer gold, activated charcoal, cbd oil, pain medicine, heat, pinella/burber. I also have cabinets full of stuff that when it gets bad I go to milk thistle, and mag 07 to clean out my colon.

The main thing for me is to get the toxins out of my body because if I don't I seize bad.

When I am in a herx, I am very emotional, and I must lock myself away from everyone. When the pain gets too bad, I don't want anyone to see me like that. If I can't fake a smile, I know I must hide until it lessons up some. At times during the herx the mental stuff gets bad, I feel like I will never get through this episode of pain. I sometimes feel like I will never be normal again, you know by normal I mean healthy. I get where my whole body will shake and tremble, and I can't control it. I had a nurse once asked me if I was autistic, I guess to her I looked like I was. The disease will manifest differently in different people. Some people have mental outbursts, some have fatigue, brain fog, etc. I get bad neurological symptoms. My face will twitch, my body will twitch, and the only thing I can do is try to find ways to stop it. As I kill off, my body becomes very toxic, and I have two of the MTHFR genes where I can't detox on my own. I didn't know this at first and when I would go into a sauna I would throw up.

Meaning when I took antibiotics, since I couldn't detox the toxins, it was just dumping them right back into my system making me much worse. I had to learn to go very slowly with whatever treatment I was trying to open my detox pathways (Hepato Synergy) does this, along with some L methionine. I also have mold illness, so that made my case a little harder than say someone that did not have these genetic issues. People have a misconception that you get Lyme and three weeks of antibiotics will cure you, but that is not the case for so many of us. You may have to look at the whole body and see what's going on to figure it out. It's not just the Lyme; it's the parasites, the heavy metals, can you detox? Is your gut leaky? Do you have metal fillings in your mouth? Are in in a moldy environment? are you under a lot of stress? So many of these things will stop you from healing.

When I am herxing my go to is my heating blanket, or my heating pad. If I can manage a detox bath I will do that with one cup of epsom salt. If I can't get in the tub I will have someone help me with a pot or plastic bin of warm water and epsom salt to soak my feet. Throughout all of this I have used different kinds of enemas, from the regular ones you buy at Walmart, to homemade organic coffee ones, to goat's milk. Killing the Lyme is very important, but what is also equally important is getting the toxins out. Some, if not most of us with Lyme have problems with our digestive systems. Some of this is because of parasites, bacteria, candida, etc. We should make sure we are relieving our bowels at least twice a day and urinating as much as possible. I also started to drink six to seven bottles of purified water a day. Sometimes I add vitamin c to it, or organic lemon to try and help with the detox process.

My lymph nodes under my ears seem to swell all the time. I have tried different things to help with this, from a self-massage, to using things like organic coconut oil mixed with frankincense oil. I went to Walgreens and brought a little plastic lotion bottle and I mix up my own solution and apply it whenever they get really swollen. It does seem to help. Also, a Lyme friend told me about Red Root extract as it helps detox the lymph nodes. I found it on amazon, works very well. If you haven't noticed this yet I am all about trying to help a person out of the herx. I spend hours helping others, trying to get them to get some relief. Lyme disease is no joke, it's the worst thing I have ever had to experience in my life.

I have mostly self-treated, because as you can see from reading my story, I couldn't and still can't get a doctor here to treat the Lyme. I have insurance, two different kinds and it has been useless when it comes to Lyme. I haven't been able to get long term treatment. When I first became sick I was getting oral antibiotics, but when that failed I was not offered anything else. I begged doctors to help me, and over and over I was pushed away or ignored. Honestly, I can't really blame some of the doctors, they were following guidelines at the time. In some cases, they were just doing their jobs, in other cases, they were just downright mean. The guidelines itself is a huge part of the issue. I will say this and some people reading this may disagree with me, but I feel that a woman going to the doctor is treated differently than a man is treated. So many of my appointments I was told I had stress, anxiety, or that if I just lost weight I would feel so much better. I have since lost about forty pounds and guess what I still have Lyme. I am still sick. The main reason I am better than I was is because as a family we did not stop, I did not stop trying to figure out how to help myself. I can't really credit a doctor for getting me out of the wheelchair. It was me being very stubborn and researching to see what would work for me.

Chapter 17: Cowden Protocol

A Lyme friend reached out to me to tell me about a foundation that was helping Lyme patients. They do one of two things, they either give out grants, or they help people in need like me get access to the Cowden Protocol. In the past I had tried to obtain this protocol, but I would need to be on it for at least six months and I think at the time it was four hundred dollars a month. I just couldn't afford that with all the other stuff like vitamins I was taking.

Anyway, I knew that with any protocol I would have to go slow. I can't detox the toxins, so as I kill I must step up the detox. I talked to the owner from the foundation, and he went through some similar experiences that I have had with Lyme, so I figured I would try it. We are now at the end of June 2018, and I am back in fight mode. I think it took me almost six years to realize that I can't do everything I want to do. I mean even if I am having a semi good day if I pushed myself too much, I will suffer for a few days afterwards.

I am not sure if you have ever heard of the spoon theory, they have used this theory in the past to explain Lupus, but we Lymies use it to describe our life with Lyme. It goes something like this; with Lyme we wake up with only so many spoons, like maybe I may have six spoons when I wake up. One spoon can be used for taking a shower, or folding clothes or whatever throughout the day. If I used my spoons up I can't get anymore that day, so then I must be very careful what I use them on. I won a Lyme contest in the winter and they sent me a box of stuff and one thing in there was this spoon. I keep it hanging on my wall to remind myself I must watch my spoons and not to use them all up.

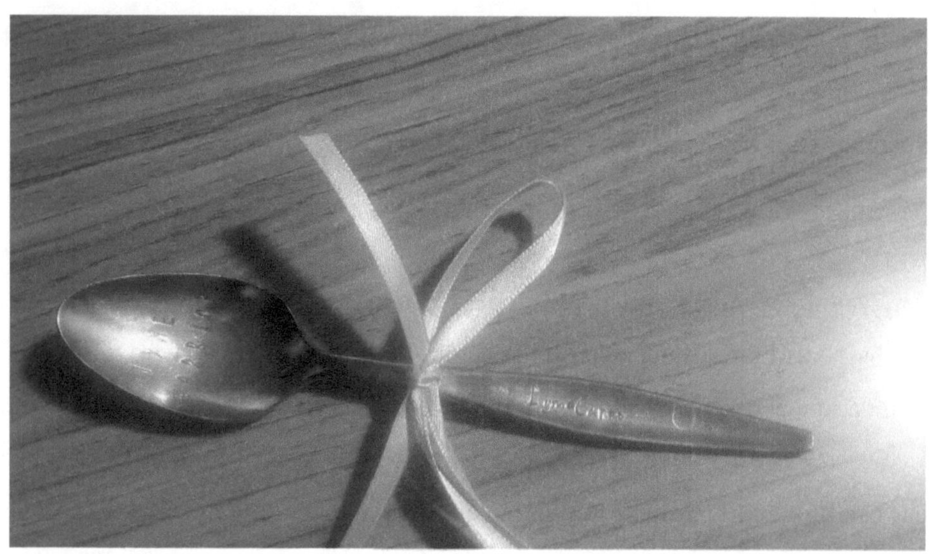

The spoon said Lyme Warrior, and Lyme cares. I feel that everyone going through this disease is a warrior. Lyme is so painful, so life altering. I have found that there are some great people in the Lyme community, and there are also some people that the Lyme has completely affected their mental state. This is in no way their fault. It could happen to anyone of us, it did to me to for a short time. These people are living in a constant panic state, and I have tried many different times to help others, but some I feel they need a medical professional which I am not. I am not sure what to do for them anymore. I do not have a medical background, I only took some classes to help with grief and illness, so I could try and help myself. I have no medical training. I am just a wife, mother, and sister, that became sick, and had to figure this out or I wouldn't survive.

Chapter 18: Things that I feel will help others summed up

Something that I do have a strong belief in is high dose vitamin c. I have went as high as 45 grams in an IV bag. I suffered some slight brain damage from a bad seizure I had a few years ago, and this really affected my ability to add. I found that if I used high dose vitamin c my brain seemed to work better. If you do not have access to IV vitamin c, you can find a good powder form on amazon. I also do vitamin IV's to help me with my energy when I can afford too. Some people call them Meyers IV's I called them vitamin ones. There is a wonderful doctor's office in Schaumburg that does these. The whole staff is amazing. Just google it, and you will find the place I am talking about. Or you can email me, I am attaching my email at the end of this book so if a person has questions, I will try my best to help them.

I also use an herbal called L carnitine. It helps me when my chest hurts. Over the years I have had my heart checked more than a few times. When my potassium drops I need to supplement it, and I add the L carnitine to it and this really seems to stop some of my symptoms. If I don't I get palpitations. As I said in the other chapters I use high dose fish oil. I use it every day, and it has really lowered my inflammation levels. I also must take medicine for my glucose. Mine goes up high and then just drops, as there have been times I have woken up and my glucose was

379 which didn't make a whole lot sense to me. I have now pretty much regulated it. I also believe in herbs like olive leaf, and I think it really helps with the viruses that comes along with the Lyme.

Many people with Lyme have issues using the bathroom; they stay constipated. I use a product called mag 07, coffee enemas, regular enemas, and even goats milk enemas. For me and for so many other people with Lyme getting the toxins out is a necessity. I also use milk thistle, yucca root, and dandelion root.

You need to make sure your body is detoxing before you start killing Lyme and parasites. If you don't you will feel and get much worse. If you don't you will experience more brain fog, constipation, low energy /fatigue, and even mood issues. For years I could not sweat, and if I went into a sauna I would simply throw up. After treating for the last almost six years I now can properly sweat, but I still need to take added measures to make sure my body is detoxing. Those measures are L methionine and hepato synergy. Also, I feel that epsom salt baths are great to help your body detox. Remember, if you're killing make sure to bind the toxins, and remove them from your body. I detox my liver, kidneys, brain, skin, every part of my body that I can. You can google how to do this and find affordable ways that you feel comfortable with. This has helped me so much with the dizziness, and the seizures.

Throughout all of this I have tried many different diets. I even went raw for a while, but for someone like me with mold illness, this was not a good thing to do. I felt horrible. I find the best diet for me is the keto diet. I eat quite a bit of meat, and I know I am supposed to stay away from sugar, but I still allow myself to have ice cream once a month. I normally will eat the ice cream and take some parasite kill. This seems to draw the parasites out, I think they like the sugar.

I am not going to discourage any treatment. I have tried ozone, hocatt, buhner, oral antibiotics, hyperbaric chamber and now Cowden. So far not one has completely cured me. Have they helped me? Yes, in some ways all of them have. I think that even though we all have similar symptoms, not one treatment will fix all of us. We must find an individual treatment plan especially for the people that have been sick for a very long time. If you research Lyme, you will find that it changes forms. It morphs when we are treating it, as we are killing it. So, in my opinion whatever treatment you chose to try, make sure you are going after all the forms if you are chronic like me. The spirochete, the cyst from, and the biofilm.

Ozone therapy

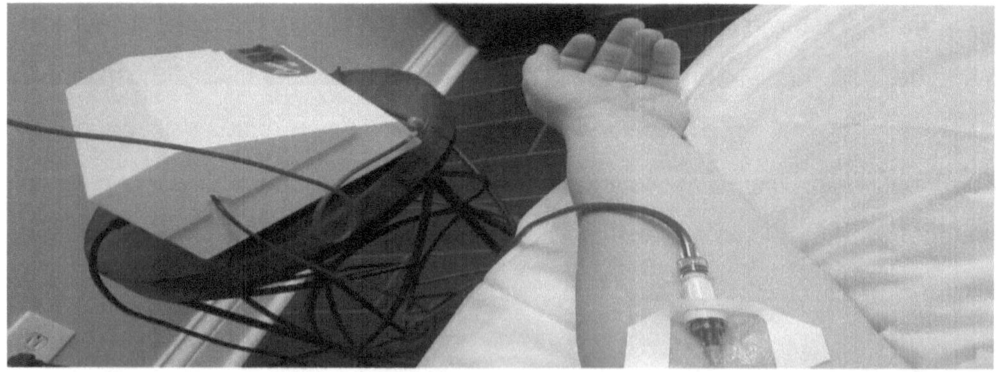

Here are some tests I think are beneficial if you have Lyme and are trying to heal. One is your magnesium level, another is your thyroid; look at things like your TSH, your T3, and T4. Have your homocysteine levels checked, mine run very low, so I must supplement with the L-methionine. If you have leaky gut your stomach is not making enough acid. You may want to investigate some betaine pepsin Hcl, I use the brand by Pure encapsulations: one capsule before each meal. Have both your vitamin B and vitamin D levels checked. Now some of us can't absorb regular vitamin b, so we must take a methylated one. There is a test called HS Crp, this looks for inflammation and if you're at a high risk of cardiovascular issues. Mine was extremely high, I was able to get this lowered using high dose fish oil. I am up to 6 grams a day. I use a more expensive brand. I use a brand by the name of Nordic Naturals, I buy it off amazon and its non gmo. A doctor can run a cd 57 and tell what state your immune system is in, and they can check that along with your white blood count. If your CD57 is below 60 it's a good marker that you have Lyme in my opinion, also this can be a monitor factor to see how well you are responding to treatments.

All these tests can be done through quest or labcop, and most of the time insurance will cover it. Another test is your cortisone. This is a saliva test, they give you four or five tubes and you put your saliva in them at different times of the day. This will check out your levels, if you're not making enough cortisol or if your adrenals are not working properly you will feel exhausted all the time. My doctor gave me a pump called adrenacalm made by apex energetics and it helps with these issues. I am not a doctor or have a medical background, these are just tests I know that my doctor and I have been looking to improve my numbers for the last year or so. Also look at your liver enzymes, if they are high you may have to really think about ways to detox your liver and lower your inflammation levels. Some of us with Lyme can't seem to regulate our insulin levels, so make sure someone is monitoring your A1C. One more test I think most people should have is your C4A test, it's shows things such as if you have been exposed to black mold. Some doctors even use it for children who have panda's disease. Certain doctors do not believe in this test, but I have found it to be very accurate for me, especially when I had biotoxin illness from the mold.

We are in 2018 now, and even though some people have changed their views about Lyme others did not. Recently at a medical facility here in Illinois I was told by a staff member that my children and husband will get sick of me being sick, and they will leave me. If I didn't have a tube shoved up my butt at the moment I would have told her where I thought she should go. I contemplated taking the tube out and shoving it up her butt. She said that she knows of a doctor that can cure me since they cured her for one thousand a visit. I said I don't have any more money, and she said if you say you don't have money, you're never going to have money. What sense does this make? I am on disability.

I am getting help with this book from my daughter, husband, and son. I am not able to work anymore. Yes, I was that angry. I am not sure if people just assume I want to stay sick or what. They have not seen what I have put my body through to try and get well. I have literally forced myself to do things at pain levels that any other person would of probably gave up. I left the office and as soon as I got into our truck my husband saw my face and asked me what was wrong. I told him what she had said about me staying sick, and he said she is an idiot, because if anyone knows how bad I want to be well, how hard I have fought to be well it's him. My kids, step daughter and husband have seen me at my worst at times where neither one of us thought I was going to survive. I fought, and I fight every single day to get well. How dare a person that doesn't even know me, barely know my situation say something like that to me or to anyone.

 I would love to say that it didn't bother me, but it really did hurt me. I thought maybe I should just hide my symptoms, if people don't know that I am sick, then life would be a little easier. The thing is I can't really hide the Lyme, I can put a fake smile on my face, but my family can see it in my eyes. I can't stop my body when it twitches, or when my hands no longer decide to work. They know me, they love me, it's because of people like her that I wanted to write my story. I wanted people to understand that this is not acceptable to treat anyone like that. My life is no less valuable than anyone else's just because I am sick, and neither is yours. So, like in the other chapters I explained firing your doctors, yes, she was fired too. We will not be returning.

If you found your way to my story, I hope that you know that you are not alone. I also hope that you realize that none of this is your fault. For anyone to get through this disease I will not lie, there is not one medicine so far that is going to cure us. When Lyme has been left to fester in our bodies, the only goal we can aim for is remission. What you will learn is that you will have to fight the hardest battle you ever had to do in your life. There will be times when you don't think you're going to make it, and you're going to want to give up. Please don't. Please keep fighting, we all here for each other. You can and will improve, it may happen fast or if you are like me it's happening very slow, but it will happen. We are Lyme Strong.

Now in 2012, I was told there was no Lyme or tick-borne diseases here yet look at the newest map that was just put out. This map just stopped counting in 2016 and look at Illinois. I want people to realize that no matter what state you live in a bug still can bite you and infect you. Please be careful and take precautions.

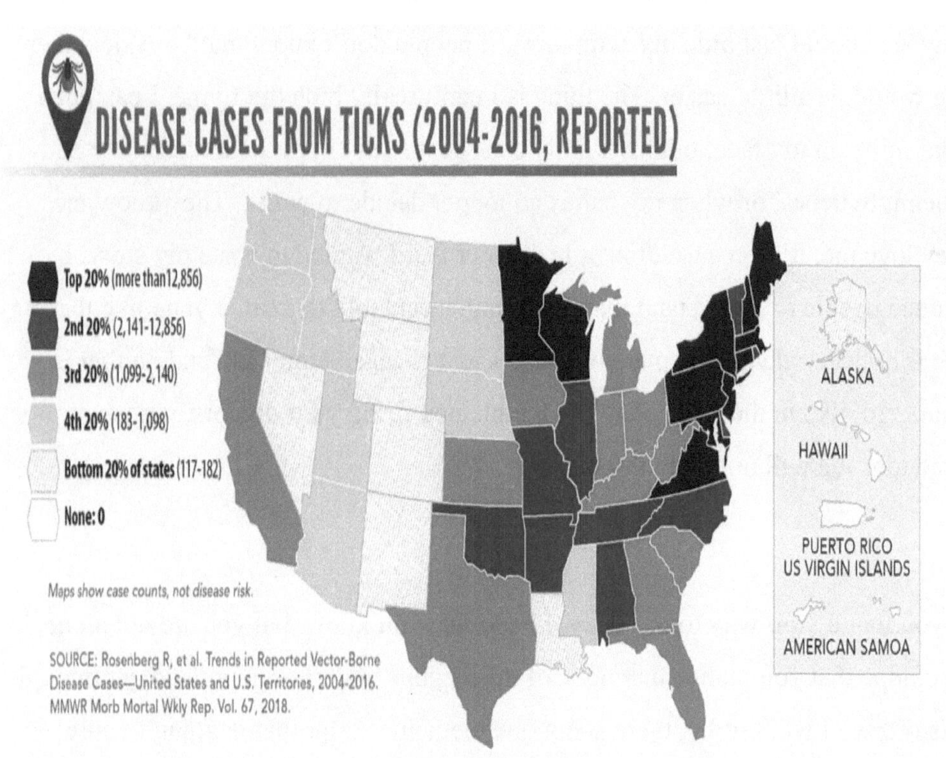

I have found these two sprays to work very well for us. One goes directly on the clothes and shoes, and the other one on the skin. I brought them from Walmart. They have the potential of saving your life.

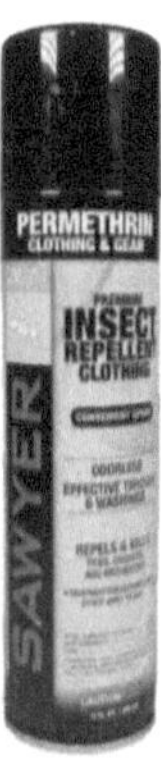

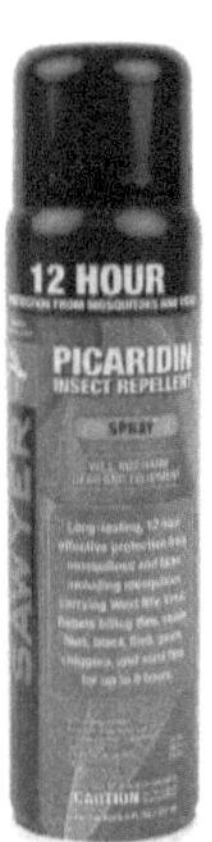

Chapter 19: The hospital and more understanding of Lyme in Illinois

On July 6th, 2018 I was trying to recover from a virus that I had caught the week before. I am not sure if I picked it up at the ER from taking my son when he had a reaction to his thyroid medicine or watching my grandbabies (my step-daughter's little girls) as the little one had an upper respiratory virus. The thing about having Lyme is I have a very compromised immune system so if I get around anyone sick, I can't fight it off. I was told this by my primary doctor and to avoid hospitals as much as possible. I normally do, but when it's your kid that is sick, you put yourself at risk.

So, on July 5th I started having some chest discomfort, at first it wasn't too painful, and it went away that night. The next morning on July 6th, I woke up to the pain being horrible. It felt like someone was literally squeezing my chest and when I tried to breath the pain almost made me throw up. I don't care for hospitals, in the past a few ER doctors haven't treated me well, so I tend to avoid them whenever possible. So, I tried to fix myself at home, I took some aspirin, some Motrin, tums, and drank a ton of water hoping to hydrate myself.

By 10 am that morning, I could no longer take the pain anymore and when I stood up I became very dizzy. Even though I knew I was taking a chance of being treated bad I decided I needed to go to the ER. I live in DuPage country, so I chose to go to the big hospital in Downers grove. I walked in telling the register lady that I was having some chest pain and discomfort, and she brought me back right away. The attending person asked me if I had any heart conditions and I said no I only had a history of Lyme Disease. Then I waited to see what he would say. He called the nurse he said 'forty-two-year-old female patient having chest pains with a history of Lyme.

They hurried up and did an EKG and put me in a room right away. The nurse came in, he was a younger nurse and he asked me about my symptoms. He asked me how long I have had Lyme and I told him since 2012. I was treated for three weeks with oral antibiotics and I never fully recovered. He asked, "how long after the bite did you get treatment?" I said about 34 days I believe. He goes on to tell me that if a person is not treated right away that they will have health complications for the rest of their life. I knew this, but I was surprised he knew this. The emergency room doctor came in, and he was also a younger male doctor. He asked me to show him where my chest was hurting, I did, and he said he was going to run some tests. Then he asked about Lyme. He asked after I didn't get any better did any doctor or clinic here continue to treat me. I said no, back in 2012 the guidelines for Lyme was only three weeks of antibiotics. I was never offered or able to get IV antibiotics.

He goes on to say that Lyme likes to attack the chest muscles around the heart, so they wanted to do some x rays, some blood test looking for blood clots, and looking for liquid around my heart. After I had the x-ray done, and I kind of felt it was coming, I went into a semi bad seizure. The lady in the room called my nurse and he brought in the Emergency room doctor with the second nurse. The left side of my mouth started jumping crazy, and they timed it. The nurse told me you just had two seizures, do you remember them. I said I remember having one, he said what happened to your face is a focal seizure. They padded my bed, and the doctor said he was going to do a CT scan to make sure everything is okay. My face looked like I had a stroke, also known as bell's palsy. After about twenty minutes my left side went back to normal and my speech returned.

They ran some more blood, and the Cat scan was normal as well as the blood tests. Then the doctor comes back in and said you have Pleurisy in your chest I have had this before, making this the like 7th time in a few years. He tells me he is giving me some steroids, some antibiotics, and some Motrin. He goes on to say they were going to call a neurologist, but he feels the seizures are Lyme Disease related and that I should follow up with a Lyme Doctor.

Now in 2012, I was told many times we did not have Lyme here. I was told I was crazy for thinking I had Lyme even with a positive western blot. Now it's 2018, and I have doctors telling me to seek out a Lyme doctor because they believe me. Every single person that I encountered at this hospital treated me very well. I admit I have PTSD from some experiences I have had in the past from doctors' offices. Anyone that has ever went through a Lyme diagnosis probably can attest to this.

My family was very scared for me, normally no matter what I am going through I can handle it well. With this though I looked and felt horrible. I know I may get messages saying people with Lyme should not take steroids, and here are my thoughts on this; If you can't breathe, you can't survive, and I need these steroids to open up my lungs. I have only taken six so far, and I can take a breath without the pain making me feel like I am going to pass out. So, I feel like we must do whatever it takes for us to survive. I must survive; my kids, my husband, my family, my friends...they need me. My little, older shelter rescue dog refuses to eat if I am not home. So not getting better is not an option for me.

I debated whether to share my hospital story because I felt it was personal, but I wanted people to know that even in Illinois that change for people suffering from Lyme Disease is coming. I see it, compared to how I was treated in the past and how I was treated yesterday, the difference is amazing, but we still have a long way to go. The day when I can walk into a doctor office pull out my insurance and get treatment for my disease will be a great day. I feel I don't have to hide my disease anymore, and I don't have to feel bad that my disease doesn't fit into everyone little box of what they think a typical sick person looks like.

So, keep fighting, if your state is not recognizing your disease contact your senators, and get other people with Lyme to do the same. I feel what is changing things here is that so many of our representatives are hearing our personal stories. As one person I couldn't make that much difference, but with the Lyme community of Illinois it has started to reach out to the very people that represent our state. Thus, changes are being made. Also, a bit of advice here, I was told by certain senators that because I don't live in their district that they wanted to hear from people that live in that area. Here is what I had to say about that. I said "I can get Lyme in one town and live in another. This is not a district issue, or a town issue, this is a statewide issue." Like right now, I became sick in Melrose Park which is Cook county, and now I live in DuPage county. I wasn't going to hear not my town, not my problem. With Lyme it's everyone's problem, and we can't stop until they hear us. Lyme may be called the invisible illness but that is only because people refuse to see it. I am not going away until what happened to me doesn't happen to any more people. I will fight with my very last breath to make these changes happen. Remember we are all in this together, and we will all continue to fight it together.

I still don't know if I will ever be 100% healthy, but I am not as sick as I was. My mind is a little clearer, and my body is working better than it was. Every single day it's going to be a fight between my body, and the Lyme. I know this. I accept this. If I am having a very bad day, I allow my body to rest. Find something that makes you happy. I have colored, listened to music, binged watched Netflix. Sometimes just taking your mind off being sick for a little while will make us feel better.

Through all of this I have always told myself I am going to get better. In my heart I believed that I would. I believe the mind can heal the body, but we must fight to achieve this. If we have the mind frame that we will not survive, then most likely we won't. On days when I feel like I am going backways, that is the hardest for me. If I have a good day, then the next I can't walk right, or I am seizing, it can affect my mental state. I must constantly tell myself I can do this, that I am strong, and that I need to find it in me to keep fighting. If you're in a bad mental state or just having bad emotional issues I would watch some funny videos, or even some relaxing videos to help you through it.

We need to remember that this is not us doing this to our bodies, this is the Lyme, parasites, and co-infections. We can beat this. If you don't think you can look up people that are in remission from Lyme. As many people that there are sick, there are just as many now getting their lives back. This is going to be us, we may be having a hard time right now, but one day soon we are going to be feeling better and get healthy. They say to really heal you must heal the mind, body, and soul. I believe that. Most people with Lyme have had some sort of bad trauma in their life, for me it was multiple things; a bad car accident, moldy house, losing my job, losing my parents. So honestly, we must heal all the parts that are broken in us. This can take time, but we can do it. We just need to give our bodies the right tools to fix itself. This is my opinion, but I believe it to be true. Just don't give up, if you have Lyme you are already a strong person to me, this disease is not for the weak. My advice is this it's okay to give into the disease for a little bit, let yourself get sad, or overwhelmed. Then I want you to get angry and fight this damn thing with everything you have inside you. If it gets to the point where you just can't do this anymore reach out to someone, reach out to me, I will try my best to walk you through it.

There are medical professionals online too that do online counseling for people with chronic diseases. Some even take phone calls. I know of one that has Lyme herself, so she will understand what you are going through. She can work with people in most of the states I was told. The last time I checked she was giving discounts to Lyme patients. Her way of giving back. If you reach out to me by email or twitter I have listed this at the end of my story I will direct, you to her.

Life is hard and complicated, but it is also so very beautiful. I want to live so bad that I am willing to do whatever it takes to make that happen. So just remember we are all fighting this together. It's not just my fight or your fight, it's all our fight. Lyme is in my opinion is the new Aids, the new Hiv. For changes to be made, we must stand united. It's just not in me to give up. Once you get better help a fellow Lymie out, that is my plan, if anything helps me I share it. No one should have to face this disease alone. Please remember that no matter how bad today is, it's going to get better. Nothing ever stays the same. By sharing my story, I hope that I can help people not suffer the way I did. I tried to be as honest and open as possible when telling it. I hope that it in some way it touches you, and makes people understand that Lyme is a very difficult disease to have. I would like the stigma removed from it, and for people to realize how bad it can get. The only way for us to do that, is to tell our stories, and hope that people hear us.

Thank you for taking the time to read mine.

Sincerely,
T.S. Banks

If you enjoyed reading it, won't you please take a moment to leave me a review at your favorite retailer?

Citations

Niaid.nih.gov. (2018). *Lyme Disease Antibiotic Treatment Research | NIH: National Institute of Allergy and Infectious Diseases*. [online] Available at: https://www.acsh.org/news/2018/05/09/tick-borne-diseases-are-rise-which-ones-should-you-watch-out-12930 [Accessed 6 Jul. 2018].

Melaun C, e. (2018). *Occurrence of Borrelia burgdorferi s.l. in different genera of mosquitoes (Culicidae) in Central Europe. - PubMed - NCBI*. [online] . Available at: https://www.niaid.nih.gov/diseases-conditions/lyme-disease-antibiotic-treatment-research [Accessed 6 Jul. 2018].

"Tick-Borne Diseases Are on the Rise. Which Ones Should You Watch Out For?" *40 Years Ago, GMO Insulin Was Controversial Also | American Council on Science and Health*, From a wheelchair to walking, one person's Lyme story in Illinois. .docx.

Walmart.com. (2018). [online] Available at: From a wheelchair to walking, one person's Lyme story in Illinois. .docx [Accessed 6 July. 2018].

T.S Banks was born in Chicago Illinois in 1976. Her family consisted of her mother that was from Georgia, her father that was from West Virginia and four sisters'. She and her siblings spent their early years growing up between Illinois and West Virginia. She is a huge animal lover. She also spends as much time as possible helping others get through each day with Lyme Disease. She loves flowers especially lilacs, cooking, and spending time with her family.

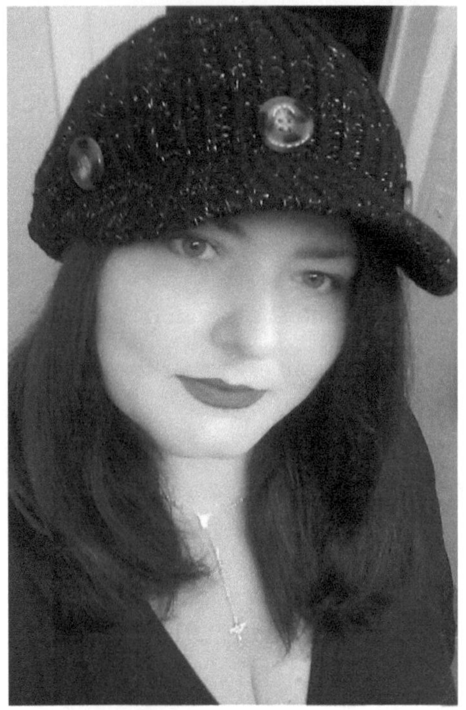

Connect with me:

Email:

terabanks4508@gmail.com

Facebook:

https://www.facebook.com/tera.banks.7

Twitter:

https://twitter.com/4mylymewarrior

Suicide hotline

If you need help, please reach out and know that you are never truly alone.

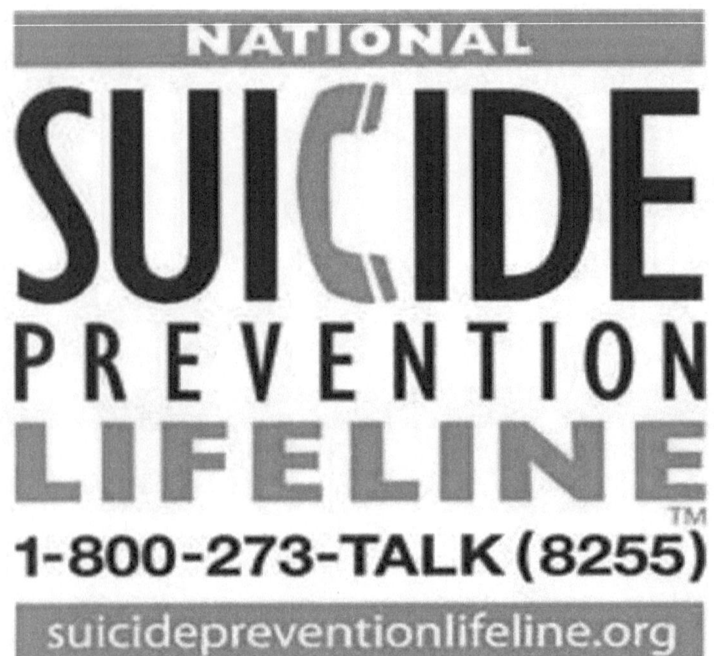